'This fascinating book addresses the use of the "performance frame" in drama therapy from a refreshing angle, positioning CoATT at the exact border between therapeutic and community theatre, and as a bridge between medical-standardized models of recovery and more alternative and inclusive forms. This cutting-edge approach embraces a post-modern, social constructivist paradigm, which is attuned to the social justice perspective that is so necessary to strengthen in our times. The book is clearly written, the Movements between the various phases of the process plainly explained, and the exercises easy to follow and replicate. The book will inspire a wide range of practitioners, from applied theatre, drama-in-education, community theatre, theatre activism, drama therapy, psychodrama, creative arts therapists, and other socially and therapeutically oriented professionals, working with groups and individuals in rehabilitation, recovery, and psychotherapy. An essential contribution to the field.'

Susana Pendzik, *Former Head of the Drama Therapy Graduate Program,*
Tel Hai Academic College; Lecturer, Theatre Studies Department,
Hebrew University of Jerusalem

'Laura L. Wood and Dave Mowers present a uniquely compelling and powerful model for drama therapists and indeed all mental health professionals. Wood and Mowers meticulously offer a manual for creating and reflecting upon the praxis of therapeutic theatre. Further, they present several poignant illustrations applying the manual to the recovery of people living with eating disorders, aphasia and chronic mental illness. Of great significance is their aim to transition from the manual to the praxis to protocols for creating evidenced-based research for treatment, so sorely missing in the field of creative arts therapy. As one who has devoted his professional life to developing drama therapy praxis, I strongly urge all my colleagues and students to read and to coact with the authors in transporting drama and related arts therapy fields into exciting new territory.'

Robert Landy, PhD, *Professor Emeritus, New York University*

'This is the book that is going to change our entire field. Laura and Dave have opened the door on evidence-based work in drama therapy, all while keeping the creativity and spontaneity that is so integral to the work. This strength-based recovery model sets the stage for success in the sometimes-elusive possibilities of therapeutic theatre.'

Heidi Landis, LCAT, RDT/BCT, TEP, *Psychotherapist and Adjunct Professor,*
New York University/Lesley University

'This book lays out a clear step-by-step guide for therapists and participants toward constructive and meaningful recovery efforts using drama therapy. The manualization of the CoActive Therapeutic Theatre model allows creativity to flourish within a flexible structure and invites other creative arts therapists, applied theatre practitioners, and mental health professionals to safely engage in the power of devising therapeutic theatre with clients. The research toward its approval as an evidence-based therapy is vital and needed in the creative arts therapy community.'

Sally Bailey, MFA, MSW, RDT/BCT, *Professor and Director,*
Kansas State University Drama Therapy Program

T0386455

'Dr. Laura Wood and Dave Mowers have done the mental health treatment enterprise a great favor. They have provided a creative method for treatment of sometimes isolating and treatment-resistant disorders. Their approach involves community engagement of clients through active participation in therapeutic theater. It is a 'co-active' approach in its acknowledgement of the truths clients associate with their conditions and the truth of building a healthier narrative with others through participation in a theater production. Their method is groundbreaking in its application of social constructivist theory — moving treatment clearly into the realm of shared experience as a healing way to construct new healthy truths for people in need. Theater acts as a vehicle to metaphorically address real life challenges. It is refreshing and will engage the most creative aspects of the experience of clients. The authors not only provide a theoretical foundation, but they also provide a concrete manualized guide for implementing the model. The guide is detailed and addresses significant and ethically challenging aspects of the work, including recruitment and screening of participants and consent through participant commitment — a valuable contribution to the literature.'

R. Rocco Cottone, PhD, *Curators' Distinguished Professor,*
University of Missouri

'With *Dramatherapy and Recovery*, the authors cast an engaging and informative light on the transformative power of theatre as a supportive force for people in recovery to be in dialogue with their healing journeys. Dr. Wood and Mowers furnish readers with the gift of an innovative and accessible approach that gives participants creative agency to reimagine their recovery.'

Adam D-F. Stevens, M.A., RDT, LCAT-P, *Drama therapist and*
adjunct professor, New York University, Marymount Manhattan
College, and Antioch University, Seattle

'As ongoing crises and trauma layers across individuals and communities, the need for deep healing becomes increasingly obvious. This book provides a rich explanation and example of how theatre can provoke joyous recovery from the illnesses of current living. Ultimately, we engage with hope for better futures.'

Peter O'Connor, *Director, Centre for Arts and Social Transformation,*
Waipapa Taumata Rau, University of Auckland;
Professor II, Volda College University, Norway

'The authors of this inspirational book present an exciting and innovative theatre-based approach to Dramatherapy. The model of practice they have created is examined in a coherent and rigorous manner that is consistently reader friendly and engaging.'

Madeline Andersen-Warren, *Past Chair of The British*
Association of Dramatherapists, United Kingdom

Dramatherapy and Recovery

Dramatherapy and Recovery offers a comprehensive and groundbreaking approach to harnessing the power of theatre in the recovery process through the use of playmaking and performance.

This manual is based on the CoActive Therapeutic Theatre (CoATT) model, the first of its kind to be meticulously documented and standardized. With its emphasis on replicability and measurable outcomes, the CoATT model is brought to life through annotated scripts and progress notes extracted from past productions involving diverse populations, including those with eating disorders, aphasia, schizophrenia, and substance abuse disorder. The authors illuminate the six principles that distinguish CoATT from other therapeutic and applied theatre approaches. The chapters provide a structured framework compromising seven defined movements that act as attainable milestones for participants guided toward producing a powerful and transformative public performance.

Dramatherapy and Recovery equips practitioners of dramatherapy, counseling arts in health, applied theatre, community theatre, and other mental health disciplines with the tools needed to create transformative performances with individuals reconnecting with the community after treatment.

Laura L. Wood, PhD, is an Associate Professor and Coordinator of the Clinical Mental Health Counseling and Drama Therapy program at Lesley University. With a deep commitment to the field, she has had the privilege of serving as the President of the North American Drama Therapy Association. Her global contributions through teaching, lectures, and consultation have helped advance the practice of drama therapy and creativity in counseling.

Dave Mowers, MA, trained at New York University drama therapy program under Robert Landy, later joining the faculty. He developed and produced five seasons of therapeutic theatre under the *As Performance* program. He is the co-creator of the CoActive Therapeutic Theatre Model.

Dramatherapy: Approaches, Relationships, Critical Ideas
Series Editor: Professor Anna Seymour

This series brings together leading practitioners and researchers in the field of Dramatherapy to explore the practices, thinking, and evidence base for Dramatherapy.

Each volume focuses on a particular aspect of Dramatherapy practice, its application with a specific client group, an exploration of a particular methodology or approach, or the relationship between Dramatherapy and related field(s) of practice, all informed by ongoing critical analysis of existing and emergent theoretical ideas.

In each case, the aim is to develop the knowledge base of Dramatherapy as a unique discipline, whilst contextualizing and acknowledging its relationship with other arts and therapeutic practices.

As such, the series will produce different kinds of books to encompass a spectrum of readers from trainee Dramatherapists and arts practitioners to academic researchers engaged in multidisciplinary inquiry.

The field of Dramatherapy is expanding internationally, and this series aims to respond to emergent clinical and critical needs within practice-based and academic settings. These settings are increasingly diverse, serving complex needs, and they demand dynamic and incisive literature to support clinical intervention and to act as resources for critique.

In this series:

For a full list of titles in this series, please visit: https://www.routledge.com/Dramatherapy/book-series/DRAMA

Dramatherapy and Recovery

The CoActive Therapeutic Theatre Model and Manual

Laura L. Wood and Dave Mowers

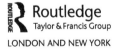

LONDON AND NEW YORK

Designed cover image: © Shutterstock

First published 2024
by Routledge
4 Park Square, Milton Park, Abingdon, Oxon OX14 4RN

and by Routledge
605 Third Avenue, New York, NY 10158

Routledge is an imprint of the Taylor & Francis Group, an informa business

© 2024 Laura L. Wood and Dave Mowers

The right of Laura L. Wood and Dave Mowers to be identified as authors of
this work has been asserted in accordance with sections 77 and 78 of the
Copyright, Designs and Patents Act 1988.

British Library Cataloguing-in-Publication Data
A catalogue record for this book is available from the British Library

Library of Congress Cataloging-in-Publication Data
Names: Wood, Laura L., 1983- author. | Mowers, Dave, 1965- author.
Title: Dramatherapy and recovery : the coactive therapeutic theatre model
and manual / Laura L. Wood and Dave Mowers.
Description: Abingdon, Oxon ; New York, NY : Routledge, 2024. |
Series: Dramatherapy: approaches, relationships, critical ideas | Includes
bibliographical references and index. |
Identifiers: LCCN 2023035874 (print) | LCCN 2023035875 (ebook) | ISBN
9780367752361 (hardback) | ISBN 9780367752347 (paperback) | ISBN
9781003161608 (ebook)
Subjects: LCSH: Drama--Therapeutic use.
Classification: LCC RC489.P7 W66 2024 (print) | LCC RC489.P7 (ebook) |
DDC 616.89/1653--dc23/eng/20230921
LC record available at https://lccn.loc.gov/2023035874
LC ebook record available at https://lccn.loc.gov/2023035875

ISBN: 978-0-367-75236-1 (hbk)
ISBN: 978-0-367-75234-7 (pbk)
ISBN: 978-1-003-16160-8 (ebk)

DOI: 10.4324/9781003161608

Typeset in Times New Roman
by MPS Limited, Dehradun

With love and gratitude, Laura dedicates this to her parents, Paul and Alice, her brother Josh, her husband, Jason, and her son, Jackson.

Dave dedicates his efforts in this book to Mary Lou, of the West Haven VA. It is an honor to walk in her footsteps.

Contents

Foreword

Dr. Jason Butler Ph.D., LCAT, RDT/BCT
Chair, Department of Expressive Therapies, Lesley University

Nikolai Evreinov, a Russian theatre maker at the turn of the 20th century, philosophized about a new "Theatrotherapy." For Evreinov, theatre was a treatment that could transform humankind, healing ailments, reinvigorating the downcast, and instilling purpose. According to him:

> It's the magic of Theatre, and nothing else, that gives you a new consciousness, a new scale of feelings, a new interest in life and a new will to live. And in this will to live, as we know, lies the secret of our victory over many bodily ills.
>
> (Evreinov, 1927/2013, p. 123)

The use of theatrical performance for transformation, healing, education, and community action has been happening for millennia, bringing this vitality. In modern-day drama therapy, therapeutic productions are a staple of practice and are created with a wide variety of populations.

In my experience as a drama therapist, creating therapeutic theatre with a variety of populations, each group comes with its own personality and character. Working eclectically with collaborators, we piece together a production based on improvisation, role-based exploration, sometimes an established text, and a whole lot of trial and error. Using our theatre skills and backgrounds, we eventually arrive at the point of public performance. Over the course, we enjoy the thrill of the creative experience and the power of the ultimate production. I have seen lives transformed with many finding Evreinov's "will to live" and a "new scale of feelings." At the same time, despite our passion, we can occasionally become lost in the creative therapeutic process. Similarly, when teaching therapeutic theatre in the drama therapy classroom, I give examples of my past productions as well as those created by others, and I share steps and processes that have worked for me. However, what has been missing is a clearly delineated approach to therapeutic theatre creation.

Into this gap enter Laura Wood and Dave Mowers with their CoActive Therapeutic Theatre model. Specific to the lens of "recovery," this model gives clear guidance for a time-limited process of coactive therapeutic play creation. Through their approach, Wood and Mowers have managed to find that rare middle ground between structure and freedom. Their method maps out a pathway with clear road signs but also allows the facilitators and group to bring their own voice and unique touch. There are a few key aspects of this book that I find particularly significant.

The most striking is the method's structure and manualization. The "movements" they outline give a clear method for group process, play creation and performance, audience engagement, and assessment. Not only is this manual an invaluable tool for drama therapists and others looking to facilitate such groups, but it is also a much-needed contribution to research in drama therapy. There are very few approaches in drama therapy with a clear protocol that allows replication. This replication is necessary to yield empirical results that satisfy the demands of larger institutions and systems that demand "proof" of efficacy for "evidence-based practice." Within drama therapy, we value multiple ways of knowing and researching, and this manual provides a complement to more quantitative methods. Though establishing a clear protocol, this book holds the balance between creating structure and creating room for emerging group process, creative interpretation, and the nuances that are vital in facilitating change.

As an approach focused firmly on recovery, this is not a therapeutic theatre for presenting current problems, struggles, or issues; neither is this a space to tell stories of recovery. Instead, the approach utilizes therapeutic theatre to focus on the active experience of recovery. In clinical work, many of us have witnessed the difficult transition that individuals face when moving from higher levels of care to active recovery in day-to-day life. This in-between space can be fraught with struggle, questioning, and a sense of precariousness. Wood and Mowers focus their work on this transitional place, helping to "launch" the individual into "the regular world" (p. 209). This launch includes a strong focus on community building, collaborative processes, and shared ownership; encouraging participants to connect to each other and to their communities.

Clear enough to be used by practitioners from many health professions, this approach draws firmly from foundational principles and techniques of drama therapy. Using the vehicles of role and story, the CoATT method is a clear example of dramatic projection. Setting it apart from other forms of performance-based work, Wood and Mowers are adamant that, unlike self-revelatory or autobiographical theatre, a CoATT production is focused on a co-constructed *fictional* story. One of the aspects of drama therapy I value most is that no matter the story or role being enacted, there is always a piece of the participant projected into the role. I cannot create a character or story without including parts of my lived experiences and worldview in the creation. This concept of "dramatic projection" helps to create adequate distance between the participant and the projected material to enable perspective and safety. By focusing on fictional roles and stories, the CoATT model gives participants and facilitators enough distance to create with greater freedom. Once the lines are set and the various threads are woven, the performers take to the stage and embody the change. As the authors say, "The medicine is written into the script, providing tangible lines and lessons to recall and apply in the here and now." (p. 140)

I have known Laura and Dave for several years and have long known their passion and dedication to helping people in recovery. I have watched as they developed this innovative method and as it has solidified into a manual for practice. I cannot imagine two minds more suited to this undertaking. Altogether, this book is a strong contribution to the growing collection of texts on therapeutic performance. The inclusion of full scripts with annotations highlighting the Movements of the approach gives insights into this kind of work with several distinct populations. Additionally, they present an insightful perspective on engaging audiences and transforming not only the participants but the communities as well.

I invite you to spend some time with this important book. While it is a manual for practice, it is also an opportunity to examine your own relationship to recovery and how it is performed for you. As a participant said in Wood's (2016) dissertation project, "Everyone I spoke to … [was] just saying how they feel everyone in recovery needs to see this and people who aren't in recovery, too! I think everyone is recovering from something." (p. 83)

Reference List

Evreinov, N. (2013). *The theatre in life* (N. Evreinoff (Ed.)). Martino Publishing. (Original work published 1927).

Wood, L. L. (2016). *The use of therapeutic theater in supporting clients in eating disorder recovery after intensive treatment: A qualitative study* [Doctoral dissertation, University of Missouri, St. Louis]. UMSL Libraries. https://irl.umsl.edu/dissertation/21.

Acknowledgments

We want to acknowledge the contribution of our editor, Dr. Anna Seymour, who has contributed to the shape of our book. Not to mention the fact there would be no book without her.

With thanks to Ames Grawert for formatting our book and Yoko Christensen for making our charts and forms both beautiful and functional.

We would like to thank all the participants we have worked with through the years in CoATT Productions.

We have also been lucky to work with many students and interns (many now professionals!) who have worked tirelessly alongside us, notably: Jessica Shotwell, Lindsey Snyder, Ellen Smittle, Cameron Wade, Laurel Elliott, Paula Heller, Dani Bryant, Liz Pignatelli, Francesca Janello, Emily Faith, Roxy Schoenfeld, Hanna Rosenberg, Kerryann Scirocco, Rebecca Coates-Finke, Anna Coleman, Rebecca Elowe, Austin Winchester, and the CoATT class pilot group of students at Lesley University during summer 2022.

We are grateful for professional collaborators in bringing CoATT plays into communities and educational settings, in particular: Maria Hodermarska, Dr. David Flomenhaft, Dr. Susan Alimonti, Dr. Hia Datta, Dr. Xiaoduo Fan, Dr. Jason Butler, and Dr. William Reed-Varley.

Introduction

This is a book about the practice of making therapeutic theatre to support people in recovery. It describes our model for making a specific kind of play, with specific groups of people, in very particular contexts, working toward very personal goals. We have direct experience working with people in recovery from eating disorders, substance use disorder, and medical trauma. But we also know that people with severe and persistent mental illness can describe their recovery as well. When we describe this work there are so many nuances involved that any patterns we see might be dismissed with the most general observations, like "Well, that's just rehearsal" or "Oh, the Hero's Journey," or "So, that's what it's like to work with aphasia." But we've been lucky to have done this work enough times to confidently create a manual that enables broad application of the model and captures the specifics of several different settings and groups. This book is a reflection of our praxis. It provides a rigorous protocol that can be reproduced and adapted to the needs of specific groups in specific settings. To extend the description and effectiveness of our work, we've included examples of the results to demonstrate how the model has worked for us under differing circumstances.

Our praxis, of course, is unique and specific to us. We are a pair of experienced drama therapists, both trained at New York University under Dr. Robert Landy, and both working in North America. Much of the thinking you'll read about is in response to working within the American health care system, and the insurance companies that complicate treatment. We are a cisgendered male and female team, a fact that figures into our results through participant feedback and observations. One of us is a GenXer and the other a Xennial; both of us are White. We are both from the American upper-middle class, but our work has taken us across socio-economic settings. We are aware that these factors impact how our work is presented and received, so we seek to be as specific as possible about who we are and what we are doing. As both artists and therapists, we operate from a belief that in drama therapy the more specific an expression in a piece of work the more universal its value.

We spent several years fumbling our way toward the CoActive Therapeutic Theatre model presented here, using the exercises and approaches from our

DOI: 10.4324/9781003161608-1

drama therapy background that we found most helpful. This is the key to a praxis – the continuous approach to a problem and reflection upon what we learned from each attempt to address the problem. This is the work of making the specific into the universal. Our expectation is that this book raises more questions and prompts deeper reflection from the community of drama therapists, theatre practitioners, and mental health providers working around the world. By providing a step-by-step guide to the model, we are inviting drama therapists, and others who are interested in using the creative arts, to support recovery, to join us in our inquiry and reflection.

Before we dive into the theoretical underpinning of the CoActive Therapeutic Theatre (CoATT) model and the manual, we wanted to provide our readers with a little bit of history about how the model came to fruition. Prior to her work on CoATT, Laura spent seven years working in various levels of care for individuals with eating disorders and trauma in Saint Louis, Missouri. Much of her time was spent asking and answering the question: "What is the drama therapy intervention for each level of care with clients with eating disorders?" Her drama therapy training had taught her to engage with clients on a continuum of techniques and approaches, moving them through distanced, metaphoric play toward a more concrete discussion of their challenges.

But work with the eating disorder population seemed to take an alternative trajectory. Her eating-disordered clients were teaching her that they needed to work in a different way. Residential groups wanted to process concrete details of their eating disorder and the effect it had on their lives. The clients demanded to know the "how" and "why" of every intervention offered in the drama-expressive therapy group sessions. Laura saw this as an extension of the disordered eating behavior, in which control was established through a fierce restriction or calculated binge and purge. Clients insisted, too, on previewing drama therapy exercises, seeking certainty in outcomes, and challenging any approach that seemed soft, weak, or "airy-fairy." Creativity is threatening to the eating disorder, which needs concrete – a counter-creative mindset – to enact its protective function. Metaphor is creativity. However, once a person is under way in the process of recovery from an eating disorder, creativity is required for engaged living, and the concrete becomes threatening.

Yet, every six months, Laura would attend an alumni event for clients who had graduated from treatment, and participants would eagerly flock to the recovery-based drama therapy group; the very group the clients had hated so much upon entry into treatment was the group many missed the most upon completion of treatment. In that space, there was a repeating narrative of the gap in treatment from higher levels of care to outpatient, and this compelled Laura to go back to her question: What is the drama therapy intervention for the struggles in recovery after intensive treatment?

The former clients reported needing containment, community, and a way to work through some of their remaining unfinished business, but in a more distanced approach that would allow them to continue to maintain their new-found recovery. They also shared a "language of recovery" that made her drama-expressive therapy groups easier, but just as powerful, during the alumni gatherings. In these early groups, a definition of recovery was created by participants making their way through the same treatment program. Basic concepts in their approach to recovery resonated strongly among group members: the eating disorder functioned like an addiction, serving a protective function; recovery entailed more than abstention from the behavior. Alumni members wanted space to share and explore these ideas together. Laura began to wonder if therapeutic theatre might be the answer, with the hope that it would allow clients to build the community they needed to help bolster recovery in a more distanced approach. With these narratives and questions in mind, Laura reached out to her pal, Dave Mowers, to talk about her ideas.

The Drama Therapy Program at New York University (NYU) was a fertile and creative ground for Dave. His internship with Marylou Lauricella and Homefront Theatre at the West Haven Veteran's Affairs Hospital had given him a meaningful outlet to utilize the skills he had previously gained in his career as a theatre director. Upon graduation, he joined the faculty to explore aesthetics in drama therapy with New York University students, first in workshop courses, and then focusing on therapeutic theatre in an Advanced Practices course. Ultimately, he helped found the *As Performance* series and served as an artistic director there for five seasons.

The series produced more than 20 therapeutic theatre productions that featured clinical populations under the direction of drama therapists. A natural extension of the drama therapy curriculum, the plays were produced in a unique setting to encounter the larger community of NYU and the professional theatre community of New York City. Dave became interested in the distinct possibilities of therapeutic theatre for public performance with an audience beyond the group itself – as often happens in residential settings where the audience is found within the treatment facility.

At the time, there were few American institutions producing as much drama therapy performance for public consumption. As a program, NYU Drama Therapy had to develop a system for producing plays while also facilitating therapy. Production guidelines were a missing ingredient in therapeutic theatre.

Academic scholarship flowing out of the laboratory raised important questions for the drama therapy community in North America. Master's thesis topics focused on the role of stage manager in therapeutic theatre (Shotwell, 2014) and theatrical design and production for therapeutic theatre (Smittle, 2017). The consistent focus on production and production values yielded an investigation of theatrical aesthetics and projection (Snyder, 2016).

Among the most powerful questions confronted was "What is the role of the audience when attending a therapeutic theater performance?" Students and faculty in the NYU program at the time were eager to experiment with several hypotheses. Perhaps, in order to consider a production therapeutic theatre, the "therapy" had to be present for audience members. Or, perhaps, the audience must agree to become an agent in the therapy, to take responsibility for therapeutic outcomes for the participants. Various approaches were applied to the *As Performance* productions. Discussions in Dave's Advanced Practices course debated the merit of enrolling the audience as therapists, reinforcing the stigma attached to the conditions that participants wanted to explore, or blurring the role of participant by incorporating "regular actors" so that an audience might be blind to the participant's mental health status. Ultimately, the program evolved a standard curtain speech inducting the audience as "witnesses" rather than simply observers, with the charge of finding value and meaning for themselves within the experience of watching the play. The traditional "talkback" became an opportunity to build community through a shared encounter, a two-way exploration of the theme of the play, inviting the audience to experience something similar to the participants' own discovery.

Sometimes productions took a concept or subject and applied a dramatherapy lens, such as *Sex as Performance* (2013). Other times we featured the work of a drama therapist with a specific population. Eventually, productions began to explore individual drama therapy treatment as performance, exploring topics such as the treatment of borderline personality disorder or dramatizing the struggle to survive substance use disorder and heroin addiction.

Subject matter for productions began to emerge as a separate consideration from the subject matter of drama therapy as treatment. While we found that therapeutic theatre forms could "hold" many different issues we also found that audiences had a harder time "holding" therapeutic material. The closer the play itself moved toward self-revelatory and intrapersonal exploration the more difficulty we had in recruiting and engaging with a public audience. Concerns about the exploitation of the performers, aesthetic pronouncements on the ability of a performer to portray themselves, and the insular metaphors that emerged in personal treatment stood as obstacles to the theatrical experience. This was expressed through ongoing dialogue with faculty, students, and invited audience members. One set of performances interrogated the use of autobiographical material through the lens of "the play as client" for *The Fading Body* (2013). Dave began to consider the use of metaphor and distance as key elements of therapeutic theate, and playmaking as a primary process for group therapy (Hodermarska et al., 2016).

At the moment CoATT began, Laura had a chosen clinical population, was aware of a real-world concern about the aftercare for these clients who are in recovery, and also just happened to be engaged in her doctoral dissertation. Dave had ideas about therapeutic theatre and public presentation. They agreed to think together about the very concrete needs presented at the treatment facility and where the literature was lacking in terms of structure.

Laura proposed the idea of a therapeutic theatre production to her doctoral committee. They welcomed the idea but encouraged Laura to consider the replicability of this type of work, as well as to consider a manualized approach if this was going to be a long-term area of research. Laura also knew that, along with manualization, the potential for moving toward an evidence-based treatment/practice (EBT/P) could be efficacious. It would not only create a bridge between mental health practitioners and medical professionals working with clients with eating disorders but, in addition, managed healthcare in the United States would potentially consider covering this type of treatment, increasing accessibility and putting less burden on clients during aftercare.

Laura had watched clients struggle at all levels of care to get insurance coverage, often being forced into a level of care for which they were unprepared. This pattern reinforced a negative cycle in which a client would start to improve in their symptoms, insurance would then demand a lower level of care, and, in response, the client would escalate symptoms in service of protecting themselves. The shift to a lower level of care simply happened too fast. During her time providing treatment, Laura spent hundreds of hours promoting the benefits of drama therapy to insurance companies, only for them to refuse coverage because they demanded that EBT/Ps be used.

Some creative arts therapists consider EBT/P to be a dirty word. Some fear that these practices will squash creativity, robbing the creative arts therapies of spontaneity and freedom. But what if creating theatre in a flexible manualized model could be a joyful challenge to creativity? Could we create a framework to play in and, more importantly, could this framework provide greater access to treatment if it were an EBP/T?

To answer this, we needed to understand what qualifies treatment as an EBP/T. Although a comprehensive look at this is outside of the scope of this book, a few basics of EBP/T will be helpful to the reader to better understand the scope of the manual. An EBP/T prioritizes improved outcomes by informing clinical practice with relevant research (Norcross et al., 2006). While the research should include several types of approaches, one type that is required is randomized control trials (RCTs), which require implementing an intervention that uses a treatment manual so that replicability can be possible. Within this manual, there are several other requirements that also must be met and evaluated by the American Psychological Association, including 1) fidelity protocols 2) cost-effectiveness, and 3) enhancing the accountability of practice. Each of these has been addressed through the years. We created a fidelity checklist that is used weekly to ensure adherence to the model. The group nature of therapeutic theatre allows for cost-effective programing, and we have begun developing our training on the CoATT model, running the first formal teaching pilot in the summer of 2022 at Lesley University, where Laura is currently an Associate Professor.

So, the journey to create a manualized form of therapeutic theatre that specifically focused on supporting recovery populations began. The requirements were that it could be replicated and that it could qualify for an RCT with the goal of having the first type of drama therapy treatment that could be submitted for review to be an EBP/T. This, in return, would allow the model to be considered for better coverage by insurance companies, therefore making drama therapy and theatre more accessible. Finally, and most importantly, the goal was to create a model that would be a stepping-stone for individuals toward greater autonomy and independence in their recovery journey while challenging some cited limitations of EBP/Ts, such as the lack of creativity or inclusivity.

The first play performed was called *I Remember Justine* (2014), and it was a sold-out public performance in Saint Louis, Missouri. Not only did it change lives and teach us everything we didn't know, but it also taught us many things we *didn't know* we didn't know: namely, that we are wildly passionate about so much more than the initial goals we had set out. What has developed and what is now shared here includes new discoveries about how the model supports people, the significance of a model that honors multiple truths about recovery and destigmatizes mental health in communities, and a process rooted in collaboration with participants and other health professionals.

We are in our ninth year of working with the model as we write this book. As of 2022, manualization and preliminary data from other pilot studies (Cheung et al., 2021; Cheung et al., 2022; Wood et al., 2020) convinced a major Northeastern regional hospital to utilize the model and contribute to its research efforts toward a large-scale RCT (as of this writing, the trial is under current review with the National Institute for Health). At this time, we feel that the book, containing the fully manualized model, should be widely available so that we can train practitioners to use the model and continue refining the process. We aim to build an evidence base for this model.

We argue that manualization and clarification of professional roles help to provide clear pathways for cross-disciplinary collaboration and the protection of participants. This is critical to the current "arts in health" movement. CoATT provides a straightforward way for professional collaboration that acknowledges the unique scope of practice of various disciplines. Professionals can collaborate with us from multiple disciplines that include, but are not limited to social work, counseling, theatre, arts/artists in health, applied theatre, creative arts therapies, clinical psychology, and psychiatry. Since we also work with various recovery populations, we collaborate with credentialed alcohol and substance use counselors, speech-language pathologists, occupational therapists, child life specialists, and school counselors and teachers. We hope this book will serve as a guide to all professionals. The book will also be suitable for researchers looking to study manualization in the fields of arts in health and creative arts therapies.

Anecdotally, as both authors have worked in higher education, training drama therapists, we have noted that not all students come to their master's programs with equal theatrical experience, particularly in directing and devising theatre. Therefore, another benefit may be that manualization of the CoATT model provides students with a road map that supports a successful process with their clients as well as training in instrumental skills for developing therapeutic theatre.

Truijens et al. (2019) and Truijens et al. (2019) noted that, while manualization is essential for research purposes, it may not necessarily create better clinical outcomes. For individuals who may be skilled in creating therapeutic theatre but who do not have a focus on research, we believe this book will provide interesting exercises and theory about working with recovery populations, and that it could infuse or support any advanced theatre-making process. Our theoretical framing of *active recovery* and the ways in which theatre can be used to facilitate reconnection to the community at large serve this stated purpose. Therefore, someone may do a formal CoATT production or may create a CoATT-inspired production by picking from the manual – or from the model – aspects that feel valuable to their process. We support both ways of working as long as individuals are clear on the differences and are working within their ethical scope of practice.

This book will provide the theoretical underpinnings of the CoATT model, including introducing its six principles. Another chapter will outline the seven movements of the model. We provide the full manualization of the model, which includes the fidelity measures. Later chapters then describe sample populations: clients with eating disorders, clients with aphasia, and clients in recovery from substance abuse disorder. In these chapters, we include sample scripts with notations about the process. We also offer a chapter with several other scripts built through the CoATT model, including discussion questions as an opportunity to consider the link between treatment and performance. We close with our reflection on future directions. Overall, we have tried to write a straightforward and useful book that has a primary focus on the practical application and execution of the model, and that includes a little Laura and Dave storytelling peppered throughout.

In sum, the CoATT model is the first manualized form of therapeutic theatre that creates a unique opportunity for replicability and measurement in the fields of drama therapy, creativity in counseling, arts in health, applied theatre, and beyond. *Dramatherapy and Recovery: The CoActive Therapeutic Theater Model and Manual* presents a step-by-step guide to creating public performances with individuals in different forms of recovery. We offer this first edition with the hope that there will be more growth and interest in the model to come. Our nine years of practice seems like a long time, but it is a short period in which to establish an evidenced-based practice/therapy, and we humbly acknowledge that there are certainly limitations and shortcomings. We cannot grow the model without a community, however, and the many participants in our past productions have been that first wave of support. We invite you to join us on this journey, and we hope the model brings you and the professionals you collaborate with a meaningful way of engaging with the recovery groups you are passionate about. This book is written in support of those individuals who are reconnecting to their community and building a strong recovery.

Reference List

Cheung, A., Agwu, V., Stojcevski, M., Wood, L., & Fan, X. (2022). A pilot remote drama therapy program using the co-active therapeutic theater model with people with serious mental illness. *Community Mental Health Journal, 58*(8): 1–8. 10.1007/s10597-022-00977-z

Cheung, A., Reid-Varley, W. B., Chiang, M., de Villemejane, M., Wood, L. L., Butler, J. D., & Fan, X. (2021). Dual diagnosis theater: A pilot drama therapy program for individuals with serious mental illness and substance use disorder. *Schizophrenia Research, 230*: 95–97. https://pubmed.ncbi.nlm.nih.gov/33191082/

Hodermarska, M., Benjamin, P., & Omens, S. (2016). The play as client: an experiment in autobiographical therapeutic theatre. In S. Pendzik, R. Emunah, & D. R. Johnson (Eds.), *The self in performance: Autobiographical, self-revelatory, and autoethnographic forms of therapeutic theatre* (pp. 255–267). Palgrave Macmillan. 10.1057/978-1-137-53593-1

Norcross, J. C., Beutler, L. E., & Levant, R. F. (Eds.) (2006). *Evidence-based practices in mental health: Debate and dialogue on the fundamental questions*. American Psychological Association.

Shotwell, J. (2014). *What is the role function of the stage manager in therapeutic theater? An arts based qualitative research into the conception, function, and importance of the stage manager* [Unpublished master's thesis]. New York University.

Smittle, E. (2017). *A guiding light: Establishing design within therapeutic theatre* [Unpublished master's thesis]. New York University.

Snyder, L. (2016). *Emotional aesthetics: A study of theatrical aesthetics and projection* [Unpublished master's thesis]. New York University.

Truijens, F. L., Cornelis, S., Desmet, M., De Smet, M. M., & Meganck, R. (2019). Validity beyond measurement: Why psychometric validity is insufficient for valid psychotherapy research. *Frontiers in Psychology, 10*: 532. 10.3389%2Ffpsyg.2019.00532

Truijens, F., Zühlke-van Hulzen, L., & Vanheule, S. (2019). To manualize, or not to manualize: Is that still the question? A systematic review of empirical evidence for manual superiority in psychological treatment. *Journal of Clinical Psychology, 75*(3): 329. 10.1002/jclp.22712

Wood, L. L., Bryant, D., Scirocco, K., Datta, H., Alimonti, S., & Mowers, D. (2020). Aphasia park: A pilot study using the co-active therapeutic theater model with clients in aphasia recovery. *The Arts in Psychotherapy, 67*: Article 101611. 10.1016/j.aip.2019.101611

Chapter 1

Locating the Model

CoATT views the mental health of human beings through a postmodern, social constructivist narrative lens. In other words, we subscribe to the idea that reality is socially constructed and acknowledge that there are multiple truths and realities that are informed by an individual's life experiences and intersecting identities. Our participants come to their respective groups recovering from the "same thing" (e.g., an eating disorder, substance use disorder, a medical condition, etc.). However, the way in which they experience their diagnosis, why it developed, and what they need to do, say, feel, and experience in relationship to their recovery may look different for each person. We hold that all truths are not treated equally in society, and that people with truths that differ from dominant narratives have often experienced additional harm, especially from the medical communities that treat them (Cottone, 2007; Neimeyer & Raskin, 2000). Dominant narratives can be defined as the stories and realities of individuals who have held a position of power and privilege throughout history.

One dominant narrative in the domain of mental health is that those with a diagnosis are the "sick ones" and these individuals need to be "healed" by someone who does not hold that identity, and who has had extensive training and expertise in the field of psychology or medicine. In CoATT, "co-action," which we define as an active partnership process in which both parties take ownership of the result, serves to challenge these dominant power structures and emphasize the voices and experiences of both the participants and the facilitators. We welcome opposing narratives of recovery and find ways to write them into the metaphors of the play. For example, in a play working with individuals in substance use recovery, some of the cast members felt passionate about the Alcoholics Anonymous concept of having a higher power. Meanwhile, other participants felt the dogma in A.A. was harmful to them. CoATT honors multiple truths and supports the cast in tolerating these differences through meaningful metaphors in the play that hold contradiction while affirming each participant.

Although CoATT views individuals from a postmodern, social constructivist perspective, we often work in and with institutions that apply a

DOI: 10.4324/9781003161608-2

positivist medical model. A positivist framework asserts that knowledge is true or genuine only when it can be proven through the scientific method. It rejects other forms of knowing, such as theology, self-reflection, or qualitative research. Some see the choice between positivism and postmodern, social constructivism as a binary and refuse to accept that the two can co-exist, insisting that rejection of the medical model is the only pathway forward. A different approach acknowledges that the medical model holds power, but prioritizes building bridges between the realities of the system in which we work and the system we desire to see. It may be useful to consider a continuum, for example, which does away with binary thinking and allows for shades of gray.

Using CoATT in institutional settings includes a willingness by all to acknowledge the harm and possible harm created through rigid definitions of recovery. CoATT practitioners focus on strong, thoughtful partnerships that help all parties meet the desired mutual goal: supporting recovery populations. Those who facilitate CoATT need to be mentally flexible when thinking about how the model works within the larger systemic delivery of mental health treatment. Although we may use tools from the medical model, such as the Diagnostic and Statistical Manual of Mental Disorders, 5th edition (DSM V), to understand the basics of various clinical diagnoses, CoATT practitioners lead their productions by empowering the participants to define what recovery means to them. Participants embody that definition throughout the production by co-constructing new, meaningful narratives. In practice, most conceptions of active recovery articulate some level of commitment to maintaining the "recovered role," and so participants in the CoATT model may choose to think of their recovery as located in a particular time of their life. Participants are encouraged to work from their current understanding of their recovered role without freezing it in accordance with any standard imposed by the medical model.

Some practitioners honor multiple truths to describe the reality of mental health and eschew evidence-based treatment. Other traditions hold only to evidence-based treatment and reject the argument for multiple truths. In this book, we hope to demonstrate the flexible thinking needed in the model. We hope those who use the model are able to articulate the basic worldview for CoATT: those we work with live multiple "truths," and the play is a container that can hold those realities while, paradoxically, we work in systems that often demand evidence-based outcomes.

We use a play as an intervention for groups in recovery. This model is informed by drama therapy, which is the intentional use of drama and theatre processes to support individuals, groups, and communities in making behavioral, physical, and psychological transformations in their lives (Emunah, 2019). Specifically, within drama therapy, our model is located within the world of therapeutic theatre, which has been defined as:

The therapeutic development of a play in which the roles are established with therapeutic goals in mind; the whole process of the play production is, in fact, a form of group psychotherapy; it is all facilitated by a therapist skilled in drama or a drama therapist; and finally, the play must be performed for a public audience (Snow et al., 2003, p. 74).

The use of therapeutic theatre continues to flourish in drama therapy and in mental health treatment. In the CoATT model, playmaking is pursued as a primary process for a group working through an action psychotherapy process (Hodermarska et al., 2016).

Multiple forms of therapeutic theatre productions exist, serving a wide spectrum of purposes, each prioritizing a different approach to group theatre-making (Wood & Mowers, 2019). One seminal text, *The Self in Performance* (Pendzik et al., 2016), identified Autobiographical Therapeutic Performance (ATP) as a form of therapeutic theatre flowing from "personal theater" models that explore a fascination with memoir and auto-ethnography in late 20th-century aesthetic, commercial theatre and literature. ATP is conceptually grounded in the intersection between performance and psychotherapy. Johnson (2016) reminded the reader that in this mode, performers are working through current issues, and discussed the way "otherness" impacts the emotional availability that differentiates ATP from autobiographical performances. Sajnani (2016a; 2016b) posited relational aesthetics as a guide for managing this vulnerability. Meanwhile, Seymour's (2016) thoughtful "Dialectical Process" observed that critical realism is at work in the self-performing self, and identified this as a source of anxiety, excitement, and exposure. ATP may include a group performing someone's story or someone performing their own story, such as in "Self-Revelatory Performance" (Emunah, 2020). ATP focuses on the challenging use of personal material and elevates the public "working through" an issue as a core feature.

Pendzik, in a recent film on therapeutic theatre, has said that autobiographical therapeutic theatre can include many types of material, including even "plays that a group thinks are interesting to them for some reason" (Sajnani, 2022). This expanded definition blurs the line of using self within performance by prioritizing the intention of a theatrical production. It calls upon contemporary acting approaches that mine the psyche for expressive material and entwines the drama therapy premise that performance for others is healing. Where the group intends the work as primarily an exploration of self, the audience presence must be considered as a helpful adjunct to personal goals, in service to the performers. CoATT productions explicitly frame the work as a service to the community, a means of connecting to others and moving beyond self-examination. The explicit purpose of creating and presenting a play is directed toward the audience. The productions claim to offer a message that is relevant to the audience (whether they are personally affected by the presenting condition or not) and prioritizes the audience experience. Implicitly, the model insists that the community gains from re-connecting with the participants as much as the participants gain by rejoining the world at large. While the material is drawn from the experience of recovery, it is intended to impact an audience with ideas that are distanced from the intrapersonal exploration of therapy. The insistence on metaphor as a distancing component in the production of the play is intended as a firm guardrail on the road to reconnection. We believe that inclusive communities value the opportunity to reconnect any fractured relationships and that the play builds equity for all through shared insights and shifted perspectives.

CoATT may share some characteristics with Applied Theatre, Theatre in Education, Theatre for Change, and Inclusive Therapeutic Theatre. These arts-based theatre projects are created between companies and their specific populations. They employ drama, drama therapy, or psychodrama in an applied process to explore and present themes of mental health challenges, as well as provide safe spaces, create connections, and deliver significant sup-port. Productions may be devised or may take on well-known scripts such as *The Wizard of Oz* or *Our Town* to help guide participants to make meaningful life-drama connections. One example is the Geese Theatre, which works with justice-involved persons in the UK and the US (Baim & Brookes, 2002; Harkins, et al., 2011) and may focus less on "working through" therapy material and more on addressing "site-specific" issues or creating productions for the joy of performance (Bergman, personal communication, December 12, 2022). In the same vein, Barrier Free Theatre (Bailey, 2010) works with individuals with disabilities and aims to build inclusive programming and theatre-making for all. Similarly, Inclusive Therapeutic Theatre works with individuals with disabilities, chronic illness, and mental health struggles together in a devised, partially or fully autobiographical production to address disability awareness and advocacy within schools and communities (Cook, 2020; 2021).

Daccache's (2016) chapter in the collection of essays on ATP suggests there is another type of work outside of ATP, called "Their Theater" (p. 237), in which the drama therapist functions primarily as an artistic partner on material that resonates with the participants but may or may not advance therapeutic goals. The conception of the therapist as a creative partner to the group is central to both "Their Theater" and co-active processes from the perspectives of positive psychology, counseling psychotherapy, and coaching. In community arts productions, the role formerly occupied by a therapist, or co-active practitioner, is taken over by a person who is distinctly separate from the group, and who leads the group with a title such as Director or Playwright.

Therefore, we argue that CoATT, with its focus on manualization, timed intervention, rejection of autobiographical portrayal, and co-creation around a question, belongs in the quilt of Therapeutic Theatre. Each of the categories of work we've described pulls upon familiar and similar skill sets, and all explore the relationship between audience and performer. Each approach may, for reasons ranging from theatrical expression to clinical need, draw from the core processes of drama therapy. But each offers a different pattern for the creation of a play.

When choosing CoATT as an intervention, there are key elements to consider.

First, CoATT is manualized, meaning that there are instructions and outcomes to be achieved in a sequenced pattern. This may counter-indicate the use of CoATT as an intervention where another Therapeutic Theatre form may be more useful. Self-Rev (Emunah, 2016) may be a more useful approach for individuals, or for groups that are coming together with an unlimited timeframe for supportive and ongoing exploration of individual concerns. Yet, the manualized sequence may be very useful for a community theatre group looking to address an issue.

Secondly, CoATT is timed for a specific intervention: reconnecting individuals to the community as they step down and away from treatment. Participating in a CoATT production will at minimum introduce a participant to the community of the group and production team, but also aims to bring a broad section of the local community to the show. Therefore, participants may meet friends of other participants, or student groups in attendance, or people from the coffee shop where the posters went up, or even prospective employers from the neighborhood. Many other forms of therapeutic theatre are trauma-informed and may be better suited for stabilizing a group to create safety or to "work through" traumatic material for processing. CoATT assumes that such work has been done in previous rounds of treatment; it is less likely to stabilize group members in acute care settings. Trauma-informed practitioners know that recovery from trauma is non-linear and the cycles of treatment may repeat and reappear, so a group may need to pause a process to re-establish safety or examine some new piece of triggering material. This occurs in CoATT sessions, but the model is intended to facilitate the work of reconnection with the world outside of treatment.

Finally, the co-creation between therapist and group, as well as between group and audience, is intended to meet a specific need to build community. Some groups may choose autobiographical material as the basis for reconnection after treatment. In cases where strong stigmas are attached, such material may "other" the performer, so the use of metaphor and the particular structure of the CoATT question to guide the development of the play may offer some safety in the process.

Figure 1.1 (Wood & Mowers, 2019) shows some of the shared elements of Therapeutic Theatre, and the way that differing approaches might yield different types of productions; just as there are shared elements among quilts, but different patterns and techniques yield different types of squares and different types of blankets.

	Applied theatre/theatre in Ed.	Five phase model/self-rev	Autobiographic theatre performance	CoATT Model/recovery through performance
Integrated playmaking and therapy		X	X	X
Therapist facilitated		X	X	X
Required public performance	X			X
Specific time point in treatment progress				X
Self-referential	X	X	X	
Planned catharsis		X	X	

Figure 1.1 An illustration of the shared elements of Therapeutic Theatre (Wood & Mowers, 2019).

Terminology Used in the CoATT Model

There are a few terms that are specific to the model, and we want to operationalize them below before offering the principles that underline CoATT. Since we believe that language is important given its power in constructing realities and truths, we have tried to be thoughtful about our wording choices without being alienating. We also have seen the model go through some shifts in language, and we anticipate that this will be an ongoing process as CoATT grows and transforms in response to those who are using it. Finally, clearly operationalized terms are required for sound research on intervention processes. We will go more in-depth in various areas in the book, but as a point of reference, we use the following terms:

- *Active recovery:* Engagement in regular activity, reflection, and relationships that reinforce my own definition of recovery beyond treatment.
- *Coactive*: Action conducted in partnership with others, in which all parties take ownership of the result.
- *Coactive element:* Exercise designed by the cast and facilitated with the audience as part of a CoATT production.
- *CoATT Practitioner (CP):* A drama therapist, applied theatre artist, mental health counselor, social worker, psychiatrist, or any other theatre or mental health clinician trained in the CoATT Model. There is a CP1, who leads the week-to-week group work, and a CP2 who leads the weekend intensive and supervises and supports the CP1.

- *Movement:* A specific set of tasks with outcomes that are both independent of the other task sets and that build toward a final production, akin to the movements in a symphony. For clarity, the term "CoATT Movement" may help differentiate when speaking about gesture or embodiment in drama therapy.
- *Participant:* The individual in recovery who is acting in or as a part of (costume, scenic design, etc.) a CoATT production.
- *The CoATT Question:* "What is a theme of recovery that you want to create a theatrical production around, in service of strengthening your recovery and sharing with a public audience?"
- *Witnesses:* Audience members committed to watching the CoATT production and participating in a coactive element at the conclusion of the performance.
- *Production team:* Individuals in the process who are neither participants nor treatment staff, but rather volunteers, stage managers, designers, family members who take support roles, and interns.

A Word About Recovery

The first CoATT pilots had the specific focus of supporting a population of people in recovery from an eating disorder. They had a shared definition of recovery that included abstention from behaviors of self-harm and maintenance of rituals that reinforced commitment to nurturing habits and mental wellness. In this construct, the addiction is seen as a protective behavior. This group pioneered the use of a "CoATT Question" and helped conceive of the model as a "survivor's mission" (Herman, 2015). Their process launched the CoATT model with an adequate conception of "recovery" ready-made from their residential treatment work.

Their concept of recovery had a dual meaning. The treatment facility had instilled in these patients (now, "participants") a conception of the eating disorder in relation to other addictions ranging from substance abuse to process addictions (such as pornography or shopping). "Recovery" in this conception leaned toward 12-step definitions, a form of abstinence supported by group process and spiritual practice. However, the treatment teams at the eating disorder facility offered trauma-informed care in an acknowledgment of the threat to life that severe eating disorders inflict on patients. In this conception, "Recovery" is the outcome of three phases of treatment: establishing safety, mourning, and remembrance of the trauma and associated loss, and the reconnection to the community at large (Herman, 2015). Treatment addresses the fact that a trauma transforms an individual in ways that can never be undone. This kind of transformation can be isolating and create a separation between the survivor and their family or community. An important outcome of trauma-informed care is meaning-making; some survivors find a formal and structured way to enact this meaning in a "survivor's mission." One example is the organization Mothers Against Drunk Driving. MADD is the work of a group of mothers who have lost children to drunk driving accidents and dedicate themselves to education and prevention. Holding both conceptions in the group definition of recovery encouraged participants in the first group to persevere in both their commitment to presenting the play (a survivor's mission) and their dedication to new habits of wellness.

The eating disorder groups created a default definition of "recovery" that was well suited to the illness and trauma they had survived. But the next groups to adopt the CoATT model were people living with aphasia resulting from medical trauma. The basic challenge to the model was a question: Does this work address eating disorders recovery or does it address aphasia recovery? Or neither? The participants in the aphasia group, just as varied in their conditions and just as diverse in their recovery as the eating disorder group, were able to formulate an answer to the CoATT Question and gave similar comments and results in the research interviews. True, this group had subject matter experts — speech-language pathologists — to help identify concrete treatment goals like word count or spontaneous expression of new vocabulary. However, it became clear that engaging in a CoATT process supported behavior change as well as group cohesion and social support in recovery. This shifted the focus of CoATT away from presenting problems, or group-defining illness, and toward recovery itself. Crucially, this shift in focus revealed that sharing conceptions of recovery held CoATT groups together while supporting a variety of individual recovery journeys. The experiments continued to expand toward substance use disorder recovery and the manifold types of recovery experienced by survivors of that experience.

The shift in focus toward recovery is so important to the CoATT model that it is included in the title of this book. Today, researchers are employing the CoATT model for all types of recovery groups, from students surviving the social isolation of COVID-19 to individuals with schizophrenia in wellness recovery, and ongoing eating disorder support groups.

The social constructivist orientation of the terminology outlined above helps to clarify the position of the practitioner and participant within a CoATT model process. We have also located our method of making therapeutic theatre within a continuum of practices that vary in emphasis on the self, personal exploration, autobiographical material, relationship to the audience, and the use of metaphor.

Co-Active Therapeutic Theatre Production

The result of our praxis is a CoATT production, an evening in the theatre in which a group of participants reconnect with their community as a next step into their recovery. But CoATT is as much a process of creating the experience as the theatrical experience itself. The theatrical event illustrates many of the features of this unique process.

The primary goal of a CoATT production is to use the production to create bonds between the participants and their community, so we prefer traditional theatrical performances occurring in a recognized theatre space where the boundary between audience and performer is clearly defined. We practice in mostly English-speaking, North American communities, so we create plays in which the participants embody characters other than themselves in styles that are easily recognizable to a contemporary audience with similar ideas about theatre. We've also found that plays with familiar structures are easier for audiences to approach while offering participants scaffolding for participating in what may be an unusual experience. We recommend plays with a narrative storyline that maintains unity of time, space, and action, because these are as familiar as television and help to ground both participants and audiences.

A Word About Casting Group Members in the Play

CoATT plays are part of active recovery for the participants as much as they are a theatrical experience for the audience. Through the generation phases of script development, the group creates roles for themselves and each other. They actively give their own creative output to each other, purposely avoiding the presentation of autobiographical material. The audience will encounter stories and characters that are personally meaningful to each cast member and the group as a whole, watching actors portray scenes that are relevant and supportive of recovery. It may make for unconventional casting, or "off-type" players in surprising roles; casting may feature non-traditional gender representation, atypical family structures, or ahistorical racial presentations. As a general rule, however, actors will play roles that are read clearly by the audience in support of the idea of reconnection with the community at large. The play will be built to help audiences understand why each actor sits in each role. Moreover, because the participants have been playing many roles in the lead-up to the presentation of the script, they often are not overly surprised by the role in which they are cast. When roles are written in service of supporting the CoATT question and each individual's recovery, there is rarely disappointment in casting. When there is disappointment over the role, the participant is tasked with changing the script to meet their needs and goals, as long as it doesn't affect the overall play as a whole.

When casting, we try to place participants in roles and scenes that will reinforce their strengths and highlight the moments of recovery they have identified as important. Because we emphasize that all written material becomes the shared text of the group, we aim to assign participants scenes and texts that were written by the group and not derived from their own autobiography. There will be times when a participant will demand to play a particular role, and this casting decision must be ratified by the group as a whole immediately following the first reading of the play or the script.

Audience members arrive at the space from every corner of the community at large; they are not a curated group of friends and colleagues or only fellows from the patient community. They may have received a postcard advertising the show, seen a poster at a coffee shop, or been invited. It's very likely that friends and family (and colleagues, and peers from the patient community) are a part of this audience. In our experience, that makes the audience similar to a traditional community theatre audience, as well as a microcosm of the world the participants are preparing to re-enter in recovery.

As an induction to the play, the lobby or reception might have information regarding the particular focus of this participant group. There may be a carnival atmosphere, a set of posters, or information booths. The induction should create an atmosphere of inquiry. There will be a brief speech from the CP1 who has led the group, explaining that this is a CoATT production and that the audience should consider themselves as witnesses who will participate at the end of the show in an exploration of the theme. The CoATT Question itself will be spoken to the audience as part of this speech.

The participants present a play that they have created themselves, fully realized with whatever theatrical values are available, including lights, costumes, music, sets, and props. While there may be adaptations made to the production to facilitate the participants, the play should unfold as any other. At the end of the play, participants will join the audience members in regular, general lighting, and engage with the community in a co-active element. Working in a community, the audience and cast create an experience or artifact that reinforces the experience of the participants. If, for example, characters in the play wrote in a journal, audience members might be asked to add a journal entry to a collective journal. If a play featured "graffiti artists" as characters, perhaps the audience would be invited to leave graffiti on a butcher paper mural on the set. This element will have been designed and then led by the participants themselves. Audience members do not comment on the production, nor do they directly address the problem of the participants. Rather, the community comes together to share an experience based on recovery from the problem or challenge.

CoATT productions generally last no more than 120 minutes from when the doors open to the last audience member leaving. For example, the pre-show event and introduction may take 15–30 minutes, the play should take between 20 minutes and 60 minutes, and the co-active element and exits should take between 10 and 30 minutes.

Reference List

Bailey, S. (2010). *Barrier-free theater: Including everyone in theater arts — in schools, recreation, and arts programs — regardless of (dis)ability*. Idyll Arbor.

Baim, C., & Brookes, S. (2002). *Geese theatre handbook: Drama with offenders and people at risk*. Waterside.

Cook, A. (2020). Using an inclusive therapeutic theatre production to teach self-advocacy skills in young people with disabilities. *The Arts in Psychotherapy, 71*: Article 101715. 10.1016/j.aip.2020.101715

Cook, A. (2021). A post-intentional phenomenological investigation of inclusivity in a therapeutic theatre production. *Drama Therapy Review, 7*(2): 169–191. 10.1386/dtr_00072_1

Cottone, R. (2007). Paradigms of counseling and psychotherapy, revisited: Is social constructivism a paradigm? *Journal of Mental Health Counseling, 29*(3): 189–203. 10.17744/mehc.29.3.2125224257006473

Daccache, Z. (2016). The unheard stories of those forgotten behind bars in Lebanon. In S. Pendzik, R. Emunah, & D. R. Johnson (Eds.), *The self in performance: Autobiographical, self-revelatory, and autoethnographic forms of therapeutic theatre* (pp. 227–239). Palgrave Macmillan. 10.1057/978-1-137-53593-1

Emunah, R. (2016). From behind the scenes to facing an audience in self-revelatory performance. In S. Pendzik, R. Emunah, & D. R. Johnson (Eds.), *The self in performance: Autobiographical, self-revelatory, and autoethnographic forms of therapeutic theatre* (pp. 37–53). Palgrave Macmillan. 10.1057/978-1-137-53593-1

Emunah, R. (2019). Acting for real: Drama therapy process, technique, and performance, Routledge.

Harkins, L., Pritchard, C., Haskayne, D., Watson, A., and Beech, A. R. (2011). Evaluation of Geese Theatre's re-connect program: addressing resettlement issues in prison. *Journal of Offender Therapy and Comparative Criminology, 55*(4): 546–566.

Herman, J. (2015). *Trauma and recovery*. Basic Books.

Hodermarska, M., Benjamin, P., & Omens, S. (2016). The play as client: an experiment in autobiographical therapeutic theatre. In S. Pendzik, R. Emunah, & D. R. Johnson (Eds.), *The self in performance: Autobiographical, self-revelatory, and autoethnographic forms of therapeutic theatre* (pp. 255–267). Palgrave Macmillan. 10.1057/978-1-137-53593-1

Johnson, D. R. (2016). Surprise and otherness in self-revelatory performance. In S. Pendzik, R. Emunah, & D. R. Johnson (Eds.), *The self in performance: Autobiographical, self-revelatory, and autoethnographic forms of therapeutic theatre* (pp. 71–84). Palgrave Macmillan. 10.1057/978-1-137-53593-1

Neimeyer, R. A., & Raskin, J. D. (2000). On practicing postmodern therapy in modern times. In R. A. Neimeyer, & J. D. Raskin (Eds.), *Constructions of disorder: Meaning-making frameworks for psychotherapy* (pp. 3–14). American Psychological Association. 10.1037/10368-000

Pendzik, S., Emunah, R., & Johnson, D. R. (2016). The self in performance: context, definitions, directions. In S. Pendzik, R., Emunah, & D. R. Johnson (Eds.), *The self in performance: Autobiographical, self-revelatory, and autoethnographic forms of therapeutic theatre* (pp. 1–18). Palgrave Macmillan. 10.1057/978-1-137-53593-1

Sajnani, N. (2016a). A critical aesthetic paradigm in drama therapy: Aesthetic distance, action and meaning making in the service of diversity and social justice. In C. Holmwood, & S. Jennings (Eds.), *Routledge international handbook of dramatherapy* (pp. 145–159). Routledge.

Sajnani, N. (2016b). Relational aesthetics in the performance of personal story. In S. Pendzik, R. Emunah, & D. R. Johnson (Eds.), *The self in performance:*

Autobiographical, self-revelatory, and autoethnographic forms of therapeutic theatre (pp. 85–95). Palgrave Macmillan. 10.1057/978-1-137-53593-1

Sajnani, N. (2022, August 23). *Autobiographical therapeutic performance* [Video]. YouTube. https://youtu.be/KOH6mRbl66k

Seymour, A. (2016). Personal theatre and pedagogy: A dialectical process. In S. Pendzik, R. Emunah, & D. R. Johnson (Eds.), *The self in performance: Autobiographical, self-revelatory, and autoethnographic forms of therapeutic theatre* (pp. 199–211). Palgrave Macmillan. 10.1057/978-1-137-53593-1

Snow, S., D'Amico, M., & Tanguay, D. (2003). Therapeutic theatre and well-being. *The Arts in Psychotherapy, 30*(2): 73–82. 10.1016/S0197-4556(03)00026-1

Watson, A. (2020). "Lift your mask": Geese Theatre Company in performance. In T. Prentki & N. Abraham, *The applied theatre reader* (2nd ed., pp. 49–55). Routledge.

Wood, L. L., & Mowers, D. (2019). The Co-Active Therapeutic Theatre model: A manualized approach to creating therapeutic theatre with persons in recovery. *Drama Therapy Review, 5*(2): 217–234. 10.1386/dtr_00003_1

Chapter 2

Six Principles of the CoATT Model

The CoATT Model empowers participants to take ownership of their recovery and create an artistic expression in service of reconnection to the community at large. The following six principles help both participants and practitioners create a therapeutic theatre process and production to deliver on the shared goal of reconnection.

Identifying the Principles

One: CoATT Productions Answer a Question

Every production is built around the question, "What is a theme of recovery that you want to explore and share with an audience in service of strengthening your own recovery?" We find structuring the play around a question provides participants with a unique and useful grounding technique. In the early movements, the question helps build cohesion; it supports participants in a necessary shift from the internal and individual to the collective, external, and community. It can also be helpful when participants begin rehearsing the play, because our plays are designed for people who do not primarily identify as actors. When participants get lost in acting out a moment or scene, we can come back to the "CoATT Question" as a means of supporting acting choices in the moment. When they can reconnect their acting choices with the metaphor of recovery (or struggles in their recovery), the acting choices become crystal clear, and, in return, recovery is strengthened.

The CoATT Question creates a parameter for the encounter with an audience. There may be some aspects of recovery that a group may not feel comfortable sharing, so using the question ethically supports participants in making an informed choice as they build the production. It also may allow a group of participants to pick a theme that they feel is deeply stigmatized in the community at large and approach it. For example, when working with one group of people in stroke recovery who had aphasia, the group answered the Question with a response relating to the stigma they face: they were the same person they had always been, despite their aphasia. This theme not only

DOI: 10.4324/9781003161608-3

helped strengthen their own recovery through reclaiming what they knew to be deeply true ("I am still me!"), but also challenged the public's perception of them and their condition.

Structuring a play around answering a question also provides a clear way to communicate with larger treatment teams. The question serves as a topic of discussion across disciplines and may help to build a bridge between the participant and professionals. It is a base that allows participants to make important connections and contributions to their own treatment.

Two: Participants Must Identify as Being in Active Recovery

The first principle serves as an open invitation to the CoATT process, leveling the playing field for all participants who are willing to answer the Question. The second principle serves as a qualifier for the type of material that is most useful in the CoATT process. Since the process is intended to present the individuals in recovery as valuable contributors to society based on their experiences in recovery, it is imperative that participants and practitioners alike have a clear conception and practice of recovery.

Although CoATT uses the *Diagnostic and Statistical Manual of Mental Disorders* as a baseline for understanding recovery, even though it is limited in providing a comprehensive picture of what recovery entails, it also acknowledges that recovery is highly contextual. Therefore, we use the term "active recovery," which we define as an "action-oriented process of engagement, driven by the new narrative that one constructs for themselves beyond treatment" (Wood & Mowers, 2019, p. 221). As we elaborate in this book, active recovery can be identified by individuals who are engaged in regular activity, reflection, and relationships that reinforce their own definition of recovery beyond treatment. Active recovery acknowledges that one's intersecting identities will have a direct relationship with one's recovery. Here, an intersecting identity means the make-up of one's age, disability (visible or invisible), race, ethnicity, socioeconomic status, sexuality, indigenous status, gender, and body size will all affect how one conceptualizes and prioritizes what is salient for themselves to engage in active recovery. This is important in CoATT productions because we ask participants to comment on the construct of their recovery, not solely the symptoms or behavioral presentation of their recovery. Again, the model works to bridge a positivist medical model framework with a postmodern understanding of the complexities of multiple truths and realities, with an emphasis on constructing new healthy dominant narratives that support meaning-making. For example, in the DSM V, the criteria for diagnosing Anorexia Nervosa includes "restriction of energy intake, relative to requirements, leading to a significantly low body weight in the context of age, sex, developmental trajectory, and physical health" and to identify which subtype (restricting type or binge/purge type for three or more months) (American Psychiatric Association, 2013, p. 381–387). It also delineates partial and full remission, with full remission no longer meeting any of the criteria for diagnosis. However, if you know eating disorders, you know that someone may meet body weight requirements, not be "disturbed" by weight or shape, nor have an "intense fear," but still struggle to have the capacity to connect in their body, to maintain relationships outside of the primary relationship with their eating disorder, to not addiction swap, or balance food. An eating disorder is so unique to each person that one must be clear on the "baseline" of recovery, alongside a detailed understanding of how the eating disorder was protective, to be able to effectively engage in sustaining an active recovery. CoATT works to honor this space of individuality and personal history in each form of recovery.

This principle helps to set expectations and boundaries around participation in the group. Part of active recovery includes building healthy relationships between participants in the show. This may be different from traditional group therapy in which there may be a boundary around having no contact outside of the group. In CoATT, we subscribe to participants building real and meaningful relationships with one another. Informed by aspects of liberation psychology, we acknowledge that the medical model has left individuals in isolation (Singh et al., 2020). Many recovery centers do not adequately work to create a community for participants around recovery post-treatment. This leads to isolation and often subsequent lapse or relapse that creates a repeating cycle of care and dependence on the system and perpetuates stigma around various types of recovery. Our second principle is necessary for the transformation of a healthy community.

CoATT may provide a blueprint for systemic change to treatment programs and communities alike. Productions may not only benefit the participants, but they can also benefit their family, friends, others in similar forms of recovery, and community members at large through destigmatizing mental illness and putting reconnection and relationship at the forefront. Due diligence beyond "relapse prevention" in the form of a mere worksheet, discussion, or exercise is essential. We hope CoATT provides one meaningful avenue for consideration in deconstructing this reality in service of building something new.

Three: CoATT is Co-active in All Elements of Creation, Performance, and Interdisciplinary Collaboration

The CoATT model is constructed to deliver therapeutic theatre in a group process and community context, so this principle provides a guideline for engagement in the work. The name of our process itself highlights a core focus: leveling power dynamics and allowing clients to take ownership of their stories and their recovery. This principle, informed by the Co-Active coaching model (Whitworth et al., 1998) and Solution Focused Brief Therapy (DeJong & Berg, 2008) states that CoATT is a combination of relationship paired with action to create outcomes that matter deeply to both parties (Wood & Mowers, 2019). As a theatre-making process, this principle informs ensemble building and many techniques of devised theatre-making. Most importantly, the model demands the CoATT Practitioner (CP) be co-active with the participants and sets the same standard for co-leadership between professionals.

Even though we are two drama therapists and have previously presented the model as being led by two drama therapists, we want to be clear that the model is interdisciplinary and collaborative, both in its theoretical roots and in those we hope will utilize the model. In fact, we have collaborated with speech-language pathologists, social workers, psychiatrists, medical students, theatre students, artists, and nurses. The work is dramatically enhanced when done together. For example, when we work with people with aphasia, having a qualified speech-language pathologist helps us add another dimension of being able to work on speech goals, and having their expertise in rehearsal helps us to work on the articulation of difficult words. When working with clients with schizophrenia, having a psychiatrist or medical student has been an asset in coordinating support.

For too long the professions of psychiatry, psychology, social work, creative arts therapy, and applied theatre have been at odds. At their core, each group cares about providing the best interventions for their clients. Theatre, with its focus on creativity, spontaneity, embodiment, play, community building, expression, and role has profound potential that remains untapped due to turf wars. There is a lack of high-level, rigorous studies for recovery populations using theatre. We hope that the CoATT model, when used ethically, with training, supervision, and interdisciplinary collaboration can transcend the divide to elevate recovery narratives. Co-active collaboration is core to meaningful change in individuals, groups, and communities that empower people in various forms of recovery. Here are some combinations we have used or could envision using (Figure 2.1):

CoATT Practitioner 1	CoATT Practitioner 2
Drama therapist	Drama therapist
Psychiatrist, Mental Health Counselor, Psychologist, Social worker, psychiatric nurse with specialty in the recovery population trained in CoATT	Drama therapist
Drama therapist	Applied theater educator Devised theater artist
School counselor trained in CoATT	Drama Teacher trained in CoATT

Figure 2.1 Combinations of co-active co-leading with the CoATT Model.

Four: CoATT is Not Autobiographical

CoATT plays are not autobiographical; however, the metaphorical material being used *is* based on personal experiences. Principle four is in place to guide participants and practitioners toward answers to the CoATT Question that are relevant, compelling, and even entertaining for an audience at large. The Question itself implies respect for audiences and the need for a relationship in order to experience a healthy reintegration.

People who identify a trauma, disease, or condition from which they want to recover cite isolation, stigma, and rigid role systems as their primary experiences (Christie, 2021; Lanyon, Worrall & Rose, 2018; Rodgers et al., 2020). An essential component of moving into active recovery requires an individual to begin to imagine new roles they can take on in service of creating the new narratives they hope to claim. Often in higher levels of care, these individuals have processed their individual traumatic material at length, but they have not been provided the opportunity to embrace and practice new healthy roles. It is equally likely that members of their community have also developed a stigmatized view of the participant and their experience. The endless repetition of familiar stories, roles, and frustrated possibilities serve to create further distance between individuals and their communities.

Perhaps the most effective material for creating new relationships and connections, then, focuses on themes, images, and characters that can be encountered in a fresh new dramatic presentation. The CoATT model insists on answering the question through metaphor. Working in metaphor, especially at this transition point in recovery, serves to help clients continue to do meaningful work while also using aesthetic distance. This aesthetic distance, which is a state of balance between cognition and affect (Landy, 1994), works to not over-trigger unfinished business to the point of impeding recovery, and serves to keep participants and audiences alike both engaged and intrigued.

Principle Four allows a group to co-create new meaning out of autobiographical material by giving it a new metaphoric representation. The encounter with the audience will allow the community to co-create and magnify the value of this new material.

Five: CoATT Requires a Public Performance

The public performance is a ritual and is a metaphoric reintroduction of the participants to their community. The importance of this ritual has been noted in trauma theory in the work of Judith Herman (2015) and has roots in several recovery models, including treatment approaches as varied as Alcoholics Anonymous, psychodrama, and Liberation Psychology. The point of CoATT performance is to spotlight a moment of reintegration in which past experience has been worked through and incorporated enough so that an individual is ready to re-enter life in recovery.

Not all therapeutic theatre requires an audience. Either way, most commonly, therapeutic theatre is highly curated to ensure that the audience will provide a positive feedback loop for the performers. CoATT not only requires a public audience, but it rejects a closed, curated audience. We want to invite family and friends *and* the community. In sprawling, urbanized settings it may be hard to capture attention or generate interest. In a small town, this may mean revealing oneself to a small group that already is familiar with the entire cast. In both cases, the group of recovered individuals must create and maintain a recovery that is viable in their environment.

An uncurated audience may be counterintuitive for some drama therapists. There may be individuals attending the performance who do not understand or may judge what they are witnessing. We see this as an opportunity for participants to practice in the microcosm what they may encounter in the macrocosm of their recovery.

For example, in residential levels of eating disorder treatment, clients may be given the directive to avoid mirrors or "not to attend life events" as they have not yet developed the coping tools to maintain their recovery in those situations. Eventually, though, the client must re-enter and reconnect with the world at large. The client in eating disorder recovery will go to an event where some well-meaning person will say, "You look so healthy, Sally!" The client who has not had the opportunity to practice preparing for this could become overwhelmed and turn back to the eating disorder as a protective function to cope. We see public performance as one antidote to these types of situations. A public audience allows performers to prepare for some of what they may encounter in the world at large with support.

Although the audience is not necessarily curated, it is the job of the CP to invite the audience to be witnesses. As part of the invitation, we educate those watching that "audience" implies a level of passivity, whereas the term "witness" allows the viewers to be co-active with the participants when considering the theme of the production and preparing to do the co-active element.

CoATT does not subscribe to a talkback format for performances. We find that the talkback can often create a voyeuristic dynamic in which the power stays with the audience, or worse, re-enrolls the participants as the "sick ones" reinforcing stigmatization and power differentials. Instead, we use the coactive element, which is designed and facilitated by the participants with the witnesses. During the Rehearsal movement, the participants design a coactive element that uses the theme of the show and creates an artistic exercise that they will then facilitate with the audience. This has taken on many different forms, depending on the theme of the show and the script itself. For example, in one production with clients in eating disorder recovery, the show incorporated a journal motif. The participants then asked the audience to journal to their younger selves about being human on a card that was provided. In another production, with individuals recovering from a stroke and who had aphasia, there was an underlying narrative about grandmothers that brought the characters in the play together. For the co-active element, they asked the audience to write a word on a notecard about their grandmother and gathered them together in a basket. The participants then spontaneously picked a card (without rehearsal) and read the word aloud in real-time while one of our interns wrote down the words and created a poem, which was then read back to the cast and audience. The coactive element can be anything that aids in leveling the power dynamics, such as bringing the group into re-connection, asking the audience to share or be vulnerable, finding what relates to the theme of the play, and finding what is meaningful to the participants.

Six: CoATT is Manualized, and Therefore Offered at a Specific Time Trajectory in the Treatment Continuum

Reintegrating into the community after a life-altering experience is a tall order. Participants must be well prepared for the encounter they envision. Practitioners who hope to support people in this task need a very clear path to successful presentation. We have found that the CoATT model will not accomplish the work of early recovery, nor will it act as a magic pill to guarantee a comprehensive solution to recovery. CoATT works best when supporting individuals at the particular moment in their recovery when they are ready to present themselves in a new narrative to their community.

Therefore, the model has been given deep consideration and many rounds of practice, each of which informed the manualization process. It is timed as an intervention between higher and lower levels of care, when an individual is ready for more autonomy and ownership in their recovery. The prescribed manualized exercises are in service of enhancing this timed intervention and meet requirements in service of quantitative research toward creating an evidence-based form of therapy. The full details of principle six are found in Chapter 3.

Mechanisms of Transformation in the CoATT Model

These principles of the CoATT Model directly relate to the mechanisms of transformation that participants experience as being a part of the process. The CoATT model operates within a framework of playmaking as a primary process of self-exploration and self-expression that supports recovery, and in CoATT this is facilitated through co-action and interdisciplinary collaboration. Within this framework, there are three key mechanisms promoting change:

1 **Containment.** Group therapy helps to establish boundaries and norms of behavior between recovered individuals. In the CoATT model, there is a layer of cognitive processing that supports containment of impulses and

emotions that may hinder recovery. By conceptualizing and supporting the group definition of recovery and then identifying a key theme that offers insight and value to a community beyond the group itself, participants develop the skills to approach challenges to their recovery with both cognitive and creative strategies for success.

2 **Exploration of new roles in recovery.** Within the play-making process, participants are invited to expand skills as group members and their skills for living in recovery. Two key prompts reinforce the learning: How is this moment in the process preparation for your recovery outside the group? and What will people outside the group learn from this moment in our play? This exploration is done through metaphor using life-drama connection to enhance relationships between people and develop a more universal perspective on self and recovery.

3 **Public presentation.** The performance of the play signals an end to the shared primary process by reconnecting the group to the public outside of the group. The co-active elements in the performance support shared experiences, a deeper understanding of self and others, and strong executive functioning in the public arena. These mechanisms of change lead to positive recovery-oriented outcomes. CoATT supports treatment goals that may be at risk in early independent recovery, such as stabilizing recovery behaviors, establishing support networks, increasing mental flexibility, facilitating connecting to emotions and emotional regulation, increasing commitment to self and others, re-negotiating relationship to self in recovery, becoming a change agent in one's community, challenging cognitive distortions with group support, reducing internal stigmatization, and increasing self-efficacy (Cheung et al., 2021; Cheung et al., 2022; Wood et al., 2020).

Reference List

American Psychiatric Association. (2013). *Diagnostic and statistical manual of mental disorders* (5th ed.). 10.1176/appi.books.9780890425596

Cheung, A., Agwu, V., Stojcevski, M., Wood, L., & Fan, X. (2022). A pilot remote drama therapy program using the Co-Active Therapeutic Theater model with people with serious mental illness. *Community Mental Health Journal, 58*(8): 1–8. 10.1007/s10597-022-00977-z

Cheung, A., Reid-Varley, W. B., Chiang, M., de Villemejane, M., Wood, L. L., Butler, J. D., & Fan, X. (2021). Dual diagnosis theater: A pilot drama therapy program for individuals with serious mental illness and substance use disorder. *Schizophrenia research, 230*: 95–97. https://pubmed.ncbi.nlm.nih.gov/33191082/

Christie, N. C. (2021). The role of social isolation in opioid addiction. *Social Cognitive and Affective Neuroscience, 16*(7): 645–656. 10.1093/scan/nsab029

De Jong, P., & Berg, I. K. (2008). *Interviewing for solutions* (3rd ed.). Thomson.

Herman, J. (2015). *Trauma and recovery*. Basic Books.

Landy, R. J. (1994). *Drama therapy: Concepts, theories and practices* (2nd ed.). Charles C. Thomas. https://psycnet.apa.org/record/1994-98841-000

Lanyon, L., Worrall, L., & Rose, M. (2018). Combating social isolation for people with severe chronic aphasia through community aphasia groups: Consumer views on getting it right and wrong. *Aphasiology, 32*(5): 493–517. 10.1080/02687038.2018. 1431830

Rodgers, R. F., Lombardo, C., Cerolini, S., Franko, D. L., Omori, M., Fuller-Tyszkiewicz, M., Linardon, J., Courtet, P. & Guillaume, S. (2020). The impact of the COVID-19 pandemic on eating disorder risk and symptoms. *International Journal of Eating Disorders, 53*(7): 1166–1170. 10.1002/eat.23318

Singh, A. A., Appling, B., & Trepal, H. (2020). Using the multicultural and social justice counseling competencies to decolonize counseling practice: The important roles of theory, power, and action. *Journal of Counseling and Development, 98*(3): 261–271. https://psycnet.apa.org/doi/10.1002/jcad.12321

Whitworth, L., Kimnsey-House, H., & Sandahl, P. (1998). *Co-active coaching: New skills for coaching people toward success in work and life* (1st ed.). Davies-Black.

Wood, L. L., Bryant, D., Scirocco, K., Datta, H., Alimonti, S., & Mowers, D. (2020). Aphasia Park: A pilot study using the co-active therapeutic theater model with clients in aphasia recovery. *The Arts in Psychotherapy, 67*, Article 101611. 10.1016/ j.aip.2019.101611

Wood, L. L., & Mowers, D. (2019). The Co-Active Therapeutic Theatre model: A manualized approach to creating therapeutic theatre with persons in recovery. *Drama Therapy Review, 5*(2): 217–234. 10.1386/dtr_00003_1

Chapter 3

Movements in the CoATT Model

Drama therapists producing plays both in treatment settings as part of treatment plans and in community settings have enjoyed the respect of colleagues and staff who see therapeutic theatre as creating lasting change for patients and clients. Many participants comment that their therapeutic theatre experience was both memorable and an important step they took in their own active recovery (Wood, 2016). Additionally, drama therapy training programs propel practitioners into the field with the desire to create plays involving a clinical population. We know that performance is transformative, and there are many ways to go about making a therapeutic theatre experience.

CoATT is a theatre-making intervention that guides participants through seven movements that result in a public production answering the question, "What is a theme of recovery that you want to explore and share with an audience in service of strengthening your own recovery?" The seven movements facilitated by a team of CoATT practitioners are Recruitment, Discovery, Generation, Performance Intensive, Rehearsal, Public Performance, and Launch.

The CoATT Model was first introduced as a manualized approach for the creation of therapeutic theatre in an abbreviated article outlining seven movements that lead to production (Wood & Mowers, 2019). This chapter builds on the 2019 article by further articulating the framework in preparation for the full manualization.

The six principles underlying CoATT can help a drama therapist or mental health practitioner decide whether this type of production is best suited to the population they intend to support. An examination of the manualization will also determine whether a CoATT production is an appropriate intervention for the individuals in question, as well as for the institution supporting the work. To understand the process of the model, we consider each of the seven movements with a focus on two factors: How does this movement support a therapeutic group process of recovery? and How does this movement support the creation and production of a performance?

We have defined the process as a series of *movements,* choosing this phrase as a suggestion of both factors above. A group moves through a recovery process, and a performance may unfold in a series of movements. For CPs, an

DOI: 10.4324/9781003161608-4

additional element of movement is achieved as tasks are completed within a manualized model.

Movement One: Recruitment

The title of this movement captures the necessary work of both group therapy and producing a play. The facilitators of either must, naturally, give careful consideration to the participants involved. Yet, in the initial iterations of the work, we didn't name this as a movement, and we learned quickly that it led to particularly challenging group dynamics that were not always productive. Therefore, we have manualized aspects of recruitment to ensure that a thoughtful process takes place.

Generating interest in the project may take a myriad of efforts. We have had great success with sharing videos, having open meetings to answer questions, and of course, we have greater interest anytime we have individuals who have seen a past production. The key factors that must be expressed include the fact that we are making a play, that participants must be in active recovery, that the performance will be public, and the time commitment of the project. If research is involved, then this is the time to also make that known. In the case of a research project, design will further dictate the manualization of the recruitment process.

When searching for participants, on occasion we would get people with a performance background who are disappointed to know that CoATT is a therapy process. This is an important point of clarification, and participants should not be led to believe that this process leads to a Broadway show or a Netflix series. In short, we try to avoid a "Waiting for Guffman" (Guest, 1996) disappointment at all costs. In Christopher Guest's parody of community theatre, the actors of Blaine, Missouri, become convinced that a famous producer is scouting their 150th-anniversary play, "Red, White, and Blaine" for a move to Broadway. When the Broadway producer, Guffman, fails to appear, the value and achievement of the production are called into question by the cast, despite their gift to the town and each other.

If the CoATT production is not attached to a treatment facility or institution, the invitation may be perceived as a sympathetic overture to performers. People see themselves "in recovery" on multiple levels, and as "actively" pursuing recovery through any number of pursuits. The first round of screening occurs simply by clarifying expectations in potential participants.

More often, however, we have people with no performance background who are fearful they can't "act." We make it clear that participants do not have to have performance experience. We often say to individuals that theatre is a representation of life, and since life is for everyone, they are welcome to come explore life through theatre in the CoATT process. We are explicit about the steps, the expectations, the calendar of events and rehearsal time, the recovery requirements, the public performance, and – if research is involved – the consent forms and research components. Here expectations for a recovery process are clarified.

Once individuals have expressed a desire to participate, a thoughtful, clinical, and therapeutic screening takes place. CoATT does not dictate what screening tools to use, and it encourages the consideration of any historical use or misuse of valid and reliable scales. The makeup of the CoATT team (CP1 and CP2), however, should include expertise on the clinical issues relevant to the recovery of the particular group. Someone who specializes in the population at hand should take responsibility for articulating appropriate standards for safe-enough participation. This may also happen if an institution provides an adjunct staff member who knows the population intimately. Additionally, CPs should be clear on the necessity of the timing of the intervention (i.e., moving from higher levels of care to lower levels of care). Both CP1 and 2 are working in this movement with participant-facing tasks. The working dynamic will shift in subsequent movements, with each CP taking a more participant-facing role at different times.

As an example of subject matter expertise helping to shape the recruiting movement, clients with eating disorders will likely need to demonstrate a capacity to do independent eating, and that they have a clear set of tools and skills to help manage eating disorder behaviors. Clients with addictions will likely need to have completed 30–60 days of abstinence. Clients with aphasia will likely need a clear baseline of language skills to work from. Clients in other types of medical recovery will need a level of stabilization. If sponsored by an institution or facility, there may be additional conditions for participation. Knowing the criteria ahead of time and how it will be formally or informally monitored for someone to continue to participate in the play is essential. These factors may help a participant to articulate a concept of recovery and help to determine a level of active recovery. The discussion of these criteria is the only determinant of participation in the CoATT model and should not be used to challenge an individual's self-identification as "in recovery." Those who do not meet all the criteria may be seen as "in recovery, but not a fit for the project."

Movement Two: Discovery

The conceptual movement contained in Discovery is of a group organizing itself around common themes. The CP works to reinforce the principles of engagement in the process, which have been agreed upon during the recruitment phase and are carried through by delivering the "Participant Commitment" with sincerity. This simple statement of purpose, contained within the model, reinforces the point of this group work. When the CP treats the manualization like a worksheet with items to be checked off without bringing their energy or creativity, the process might become reminiscent of Dialectical Behavioral Therapy worksheets. Therefore, we encourage CPs to embody these commitments in a way that is genuine for them and the group. Additionally, the CP works to support participants in building rapport and defining active recovery, and to highlight moments when the group is demonstrating active recovery through process commentary beyond the manualization.

In terms of play-making, during this movement, we are working toward choosing a theme of recovery that we can explore in this production, as well as share with a public audience in service of strengthening recovery. As a starting point, CP1 will lead participants through tasks that initially deal with some level of personal and autobiographical material. In early sessions, the manualized tasks owe a debt to Landy's (1994) Role Method. The first exercise in which participants play their recovery through monologue is particularly important as it presents the concept of recovery through multiple roles. It also begins scaffolding, creating manageable steps, for the group to work through metaphor. When recovery is embodied as Recovery, the role serves as a projective object for the participant to discover areas of strength and growth (Landy, 1994).

In addition to Landy (1994), a nod also goes to Richard Schwartz's (1995) Internal Family System (IFS) Model, which asserts that "maladaptive behaviors" can instead be conceptualized as protective functions. CoATT exercises, especially "play your recovery" encourage practitioners and participants to consider "maladaptive" or "compensatory" behaviors as protective functions that someone developed as their only option given the circumstances in their life at that point. For example, a participant might – in the role of "Recovery" – characterize their addiction as a monster to be killed off. When the group gets to interview "Recovery," they may want to consider the IFS concept of protection. Is the addiction really a monster that needs to be killed off? Or was addiction a misguided monster that was doing the best it could, given the circumstances, and needed help in transforming? Ultimately, the participant decides how they see their Recovery in relationship to whatever we are exploring at hand. We do find, though, that at least the offer of a compassionate, curious approach opens dramatic avenues of support for that part of themselves that they are transforming into a new role in their active recovery (Schwartz & Sweezy, 2019).

The "play your Recovery" exercise also supports participants in looking at intersections in their own recovery alongside another participant's recovery. This is an important developmental phase that some individuals in recovery need to work through as they may still be holding onto the belief that their addiction, struggle, trauma, or other experience is so incredibly unique that *no one* else could possibly understand their story, in turn leaving individuals alone in shame and isolation. In these instances, the addiction or trauma suffered often has become a core part of the individual's identity; a protective badge to wear as a way of being known and seen in the world. While the individual's story is certainly unique to them, actively blocking others from relating is a noteworthy relational pattern.

For example, we worked with a participant with an eating disorder that developed, in part, as a protective function to create separation from her mother with whom she was enmeshed. The participant could only find connection and have her needs met with her mother by being a narcissistic extension of her, meaning every action she did had to be seen in a favorable light by her mother, who saw her daughter and herself as one and the same. One protective function of her eating disorder was that it provided separation and a way for her to claim her own identity: "I am different from you, mom; I have an eating disorder; see me! I am NOT you!" When she entered treatment, she felt threatened when others tried to relate to her by sharing what they had in common. Rather than hearing the genuine desire of fellow group members looking to connect, she felt trapped in the way she did with her mother. She would assert to the group that her eating disorder was "much worse" than anyone else's. As further protection, she would make this assertion through rage, furious that others dare to try to relate to her. Internally and privately in individual therapy, however, she would report feeling suffocated, unseen, and sad. These polarized feelings left her confused; she was relieved because she was finally able to claim space that was her own, but she also felt profoundly lonely in the world and wished she could claim space without resorting to rage. So, she would return to the eating disorder and isolation, fearing that it was the only action she could take to soothe and regulate her. She worked through this in higher levels of care and began to understand the ways the attachment trauma had fueled her need to hold onto her eating disorder as a way of trying to individuate and be seen. In her conception of active recovery from an eating disorder, she wanted to have compassion for the way the eating disorder served as a protector while recognizing how it kept her from forming meaningful relationships. For her, active recovery was sharing in the universality of recovery *and* looking for new and healthy ways to individuate and cultivate her authentic self and voice. CoATT is timed to give clients like this the real-world practice of discovering, playing with, and claiming new aspects of themselves with, and in relationship to, the other. Although she struggled in Discovery around finding the common theme with the group, she also had a reparative experience, being both connected in the theme the group identified and also having space to experience the theme in her own unique way. Through CoATT she could both relate to others and still stand proud in her own voice and experience, a very different experience than the day-to-day enmeshment with her mother.

Typically, Session Two rallies the group to find the courage to name the aspects of recovery that are still challenging, and it gives them a way to work on it. The exercises are executed with aesthetic distance, a state in which affect and cognition are in harmony, providing a pathway to make the difficult more tolerable emotionally and psychologically. The group makes the following statement to each other: "We commit to working towards a meaningful theme that will benefit our recovery and the community at large." When participants can pick a theme that is in service of strengthening recovery, it drives the show and character choices and heightens the meaning-making in the play process.

People in recovery have often been locked into the stigma around their struggle (i.e., primarily being seen as the aphasia or the addiction, rather than being seen as a whole person). Treatment as usual, as well as the institutions that offer treatment, may systematically reinforce this perception. In Discovery, we dismantle and re-story the narrative on the micro and macro levels. We also see that people have more meaningful and lasting recoveries when they can become agents of change in their own communities. Co-creation in the Discovery phase foreshadows the co-creation of change in a community that may result from creating a performance in service of self and others.

The Discovery movement contains a sequence of exercises in which participants begin with more autobiographical work in preparation for more metaphorical work. This eventually progresses to scene work, and then to group scenes. So far, participants have done monologues from autobiographical material in a previous session, and now generate another brief monologue before entering a dialogue with CP1. Participants do not use the exercises for self-exploration, but they apply them to the discovery of a theme and exploration of a concept outside themselves. The subject matter is familiar and may have personal meaning, but CP1 focuses the work on an external construct, with the explicit reminder and commitment to work in service of an audience that will attend a performance at a later date.

In the "Future Talk Show" exercise, the participants imagine that it is five years from now, and they are fully recovered. CP1 facilitates this session and leads the participants in the creation of a character that is in this new reality. The group plays the audience and gets to ask questions about how the person came to be so successful in their recovery. CP1 can also use this time to ask questions about areas that the person may be struggling with.

For example, Rhonda, in the substance use recovery group, is struggling with feeling like using heroin is a quicker fix than having to sit with emotions – and therefore, recovery feels hard to maintain. The Future Talk Show Host (CP1) may ask, "So, Rhonda, something that we know is that in the early stages of recovery, learning to do things without someone's drug of choice is really hard. Five years ago – I know that was a struggle for you. How did you get to the place where it isn't as much of a struggle?" This exercise provides the participants an opportunity to start working on the concept of being in a role, and the paradox that when you play a role it is both you and not you (Landy, 1994). Participants typically enjoy the dynamic of the "role of recovered person" because they know they can't break character and must come up with something clever. Many times, they also play with the subtext of the dynamic. In this example, Rhonda rolls her eyes and laughs; she must use dramatic reality to help her answer the question she is struggling with in the present, but discover the wisdom from the role of her future self. "Well, Laura, that was a really hard thing for me, but I participated in this thing called the CoATT model and this really annoying leader and wacky group somehow helped me work through it." The group then breaks into a roar of laughter. CP1 can find ways to infuse their creativity and playfulness into this exercise both in service of modeling playfulness for the group and to build ego strength and courage.

Movement Three: Generation

The goal of Generation is to simply do that: generate material. This movement is about embracing the notion of creating, and the vehicle is scene work. Participants understand this, as it is reflected in the commitment, "We commit to exploring the selected theme through role, story, and metaphor … ." They know they are responsible for a script, and the performance date looms in the distance. CP1 balances this tension with wisdom about the creative process, and perhaps shares an insight from successful, working artists. For example, as an American journalist and host of *This American Life* on National Public Radio, Ira Glass has described:

> All of us who do creative work … we get into it because we have good taste. … But there's a gap. [F]or the first couple years you make stuff, what you're making isn't so good. … But your taste, the thing that got you into the game, your taste is still killer. And your taste is good enough that you can tell that what you're making is kind of a disappointment to you. … A lot of people never get past that phase; a lot of people at that point, they quit. [But] most everybody I know who does interesting, creative work, they went through a phase of years of [this]. … Everybody goes through that. We all go through this. [Y]ou gotta know it's totally normal and the most important thing, possible thing you could do, is do a lot of work. Do a huge volume of work. Put yourself on a deadline so that every week or every month you know you're gonna finish one story. … It is only by actually going through a volume of work that you're actually going to catch up and close that gap, and your work you're making will be as good as your ambitions. (Warphotography, 2009)

Invoking and embodying this mentality is essential because, as Mr. Glass points out, a lot of the participants are excited and creative individuals, but they haven't had the time to cultivate an artist identity because they have been protected by their addiction, medical complication, or some other factor. When participants enter the CoATT process, they may struggle to formulate any ideas, or they may come up with one singular idea and become overly attached to it. Just like recovery and trying many strategies to be in the world differently, creating is the same; we draw these parallels to infuse the process and recovery. We give clear anticipatory guidance around this at the start of Generation. Facilitators practice a mixture of side-coaching acting skills along with supportive therapeutic intervention as participants master the skills of embodiment, improvisation, creating characters, and responding in the moment. The group keeps its attention on generating new approaches to the material and the performance. A personal reflection taken from a prescribed homework assignment becomes a new and different piece with simple adjustments such as "play it loud" or "do it as a frog." Participants soon incorporate the ability to keep approaching their recovery with a creative mindset and not give in to frustration. In addition, anytime a question comes up during Generation, we ground ourselves by coming back to the theme: What do we want the audience to know, and how will it support our active recovery?

The work in Generation begins with participants being offered a list of character ideas, which CP1 and CP2 have prepared ahead of time. Drama therapists may draw from Landy's (1996) Role Taxonomy, or, when appropriate, draw from those who have done variations on Landy's work, such as Stevens' (2023) Black American Role Taxonomy. Counselors who have theatre training may find themselves working with Jung's archetypes, theatre practitioners may draw from stock characters such as those in the Commedia dell'arte or the boulevard comedies of Moliere. Participants may add characters to the list from familiar television shows or film, and from other media sources like Manga or comic books, or role-playing games (RPGs). CP1 works to make contemporary character suggestions accessible without limiting a wide range of options. For example, if the character is a specific famous person such as Lady Gaga or The Rock, CP1 can prompt for a general descriptor such as Rock Star or Movie Star. In the case of Duane "The Rock" Johnson, the group may gain several roles including Wrestler, Superhero, Movie Star, Leading Man, or Millionaire.

The sessions build on comfort with speaking in monologue, but give dimension to characters through questions such as, "How does this role walk when it's tired? Excited? Inspired?" Participants think about how feelings states, an important aspect of a successful final performance, perform in the body. Sessions are time-limited so, after exploring two roles in the space, participants choose the one that they felt more drawn to working with. A list of potential scene starters, generated by CP1 and CP2, is offered to participants and improvised. The scene suggestions will be relevant to the themes being explored and will be open-ended to encourage true ownership by the participants when improvising. The list should not dictate action or outcomes for any scene.

Generation continues for several weeks following the same structure. Typically, the Intensive movement starts in week six, but if more weeks are needed or are planned in the Generation movement, the above exercises continue to repeat. We rarely find that people need more than the five weeks to head into the weekend Intensive; in fact, we have done discovery and generation in three weeks with some more-skilled groups, or in seasoned groups that may be working on their second production.

CP1 captures all scenes and characters in rehearsal notes, and this mate-rial, along with all previous creative session notes and homework is handed off to CP2. In weekly meetings, the team meets without the participants to clarify themes and learn the material. This will be the raw material of the first draft script, so cataloging the output of the group is critical. CP1 may reflect this dynamic to the participants with the reminder that all material is shared and becomes "property of the group," and that we are in a process of "looking for the best of our work that answers our question." This creates a framework for the participants to take co-ownership of the material and the finished product. It also becomes a rationale and the foundation for shared decision-making, expressing preferences, sharing praise, and tolerating adjustments.

Movement Four: The Intensive

The performance Intensive is a time for shifting the focus of the group toward making and presenting a play, and while the participants already have been thinking that way in previous sessions, they are now focusing on a specific play. The Intensive should produce an ensemble that is specific to a script, and a script for the specific ensemble in the room. We focus on acting skills training and empowering participants to authentically relate to, as well as connect – on and off the stage – with one another. The Intensive is usually held over three consecutive days: a Friday night, an eight-hour day on Saturday, and a half a day on Sunday. Ideally, on Sunday the script is presented and read for the first time. Depending on the needs of the group, however, this can be altered. For example, with clients with aphasia, the three days needed to be spread out to help with the natural fatigue that accompanies the condition. So, although the Intensive movement is presented as three sessions (labeled a, b, and c), it may be most helpful to look at the tasks and workload as the commitment from participants and CP2. In our experience, sessions 6a and 6b may be collapsed and shortened, but session 6c is a standalone meeting that must be held according to the model.

Since the focus of this movement is a script, the tasks are aimed at producing the document during the Intensive period, and because CP1 has been sharing rehearsal notes and homework with CP2, the team will have identified an approach to the play together. Careful organization will have ensured that the earlier sessions may have generated the exact scenes and monologues that will become the script, and the Intensive program would be used to refine the draft. In more wide-ranging exploratory early sessions, ideas, and themes, as well as characters, will have emerged that inform the work in the Intensive. Since CP2 will lead this movement, they must develop a program for the sessions in advance. All the material that has been generated thus far becomes the property of the group. Script development may take the form of extended improvisations, script interpretation of material written by other group members, more comprehensive character exploration, music-making, song, dance, or movement.

There is no substitute for an extensive body of experience devising and directing plays. We have found, however, that the approach suggested in our manual gives any CP2 a strong guideline for using this time productively. In the first session, practicing basic terminology and staging allows a CP2 to assess the comfort and previous experience of participants. A second set of exercises allows the group to gain comfort by creating, improvising, and performing with each other in the presence of a new figure: CP2. Finally, to introduce the work sessions that will follow, the group should present the material they are already comfortable with and proud to perform for the newcomer. CP2 must model a receptive and collaborative stance for the work of the group. Appropriate feedback includes, "Thank you. That presentation made me feel ...," and, more importantly, "Thank you. That piece makes me want to ask this question: 'what if ...?'." Though we are focused on the theatre-making, CP2 continues and extends the therapeutic presence of CP1.

Session 6b is intended to be the lengthiest. Here, CP2 supports the group in developing the work that will be presented. CP2 must have a work plan for this session that has clear goals toward script development. This means arriving with a set of ideas for a fully realized production based on the material of previous sessions, as well as with the introduction to the group in session 6a. A smart work plan will include an exploration of the material that is most relevant to the theme while continuing to engage collaboratively with the participants, which is most likely to appear in a final form. This is another area where having two facilitators in the process is essential, as working ideas move through an iterative process involving co-facilitators and group members all become more attuned to one another. As in any creative brainstorming process, any idea is welcomed in its first iteration and appreciated as an effort toward the success of the group. Improvisation and on-the-spot writing exercises may enrich pieces that already exist. Scenes and monologues may be extended, cut, or interpolated. CP2 invites the group to make these discoveries "on their feet" and through "trying it out," rather than by puzzling it out on the page or at the keyboard (the keyboard will show up later).

While any technique from the wide range of drama therapy or applied theatre methods is valuable during the Intensive rehearsal, practitioners should plan to create a linear narrative using unified time, space, and action when confronting the audience in production. Within the manualized limitations of the Intensive, any approach to playmaking is welcome.

No amount of focus on "the work" should dislodge the primary focus of the CoATT model: supporting individuals in their recovery as they move into their community. The participants and CP2 will be well versed in reflecting on each moment of the process with the questions: "How is this moment like recovery?" and "What are we learning through this exploration that can support us in recovery?"

At the end of the Intensive, CP2 creates a skeletal script and presents it to the cast. This typically happens in an overnight writing session. We strongly encourage CP1 and CP2 to create the script together; it is wisest to schedule session 6c much later in the day if possible. The team should also prepare for the practical implications of this turnaround: there must be access to a computer and a printer so that everyone will have a script the following day. Different teams approach the writing differently, but there are two key factors here: 1) every element of the script, including the actual words on the page, should come from the work of the participants, and 2) the script should be a direct demonstration of the theme chosen by the participants. For example, if the theme in recovery is "slow down," the script must be an overt exploration of going slower or suffering from going too fast. If the theme is "recovery is scary, but you must keep taking the actions anyway," the script will directly reflect the discovery of courage, or the necessity of action.

These stories will not be stories of recovery from a condition, trauma, or a disease attributable to the participants. A presentation by a substance use disorder group will not be a play about alcoholism, nor will a play about recovery from eating disorders be about bingeing or purging food. The material generated from early sessions, as well as from the Intensive, will have taken a creative and metaphoric approach to the subject of recovery. So, the play itself will most likely lead CP2 toward a strong story with a relevant theme.

CP2 will use the scenes and monologues that were both written by the participants and amended in the Intensive to create a script. It is important that recognizable passages remain intact, as they were submitted. All material is available for group use, though, so monologues may be created by stitching together a variety of pieces, or by condensing a scene. Dialogue from differing scenes can be cut together to make richer and more dynamic exchanges. Lines, speeches, and characters can be re-assigned. CP1 advises CP2 on the therapeutic value of assigning scenes and speeches, or of creating dynamics that will enrich the recovery of individual participants. For example, one participant in a CoATT group dedicated to recovery from eating disorders needed to work on building a social life without the old friends that triggered old behaviors. So, in the play, he had a scene where he literally left a destructive friend behind. In another play, a participant had lost her mother in real life, and since she had longed for an opportunity to say certain things to her mother, her character had a speech in the play clearing the air before reconciling with a mother figure in the play.

The key to writing the script overnight is preparation. Just as preparation for the Intensive included familiarity with the scenes and monologues already generated, the writing of the play will benefit from some forethought. CP2 may be generating a list of theatrical tropes that mirror the recovery of the participants, or they may be thinking of plays that express a similar theme. CP2 may be thinking of ensemble casts on television or in film who have similar characters to the participants and their characters. Inspiration is found in styles, genres, catalogs of painting, epochs of history, legends, tall tales, folklore, and religion. No cheat sheet will suffice to prepare CP2, except for a list of images and ideas that inspire them.

Some specific examples from CoATT productions may suggest one way that CP2 can prepare to write. Consider several titles from the library of CoATT production scripts (some of which are included later in this book). The reunion of long-lost twins with their mother in *Paths of the Prism* borrows from Shakespeare's *Comedy of Errors*, but the journey of one character in search of her "heart" is inspired by Viola in *Twelfth Night*. In *Twin Falls*, Miss Waits' monologue while she sweeps the floor alone is inspired by Young Cosette in *Les Miserables*; *I Remember Justine* is a pastiche of scenes that include inspiration from the Apostle Paul being struck blind on the road to Damascus, a kidnapping from Stevenson's *Treasure Island*, and a circus act from Ringling Brothers clowns that were all stitched together with a piece of staging inspired by Mary Zimmerman's *Metamorphosis*. These images and scenes made their way into the Intensive, were transformed by the participants, were made relevant to the themes of recovery, and were then written into the script for a first draft.

CoATT recommends that the story of the play follows a simple unity of time, space, and action. Most CoATT plays have a linear narrative that moves forward through time, characters that are recognizable as they change, and logical cause and effect. There are several reasons for this approach. First, the ultimate goal is to create a connection with an audience through a public performance. This connection is most likely to occur when the dramatic form is recognizable and accessible. Second, the goal for participants is to deliver a performance that lets them feel proud, connected, and capable as they reconnect to their community. The simpler narrative structures support success because logical progression is intuitive and more predictable. Another consideration is reality testing; in straightforward texts with a cohesive reality, it is easier to enter and exit dramatic reality. For example, it is easy to lose oneself, literally, in long passages of dense poetry that slip in and out of time. It is much easier to say, "Now I am the King and the father of a Princess," or "now I am myself, a participant in the CoATT group." Finally, it may be easier to take personal and interpersonal risks in a play that feels familiar and comfortable.

This is not to say that a CoATT production must be a situational comedy or must be a strictly naturalistic and realistic story. CoATT plays have gods and monsters, pirates and sorcerers, angels, and artists, as well as nuclear families and chosen families. We play scenes in Starbucks and tableaus in Olympus. The most successful scripts give simple, grounded explanations for what is happening on stage and preserve a logic that allows for the suspension of disbelief. These guidelines are especially important to bear in mind when sharing the script with the participants for the first time. Expect them to say, "I don't get it," "I don't believe it," and "that would never happen." The CPs encourage this resistance and work both with it and through it to empower participants to shape their experience. In Rehearsal, they will learn to collaborate toward a solution and to take ownership of problem-solving. The script is a vehicle to therapeutic theatre as a primary process in recovery; we learn skills for living by learning skills for making the production.

The final activity of the Intensive is to read through the script as a cast and discuss how the participants take ownership of the narrative of the play. The cast response often projects feelings of disappointment, fear that the message isn't clear, and, at times, anger. It may also involve feelings of delight, surprise, and humor. CP2 enlists all responses to motivate the cast in a co-created writing process so they can complete a working script in the rehearsal movement. CP1 is present to make the commitment with participants, and also comes in to remind the cast of their participant commitment for Rehearsal at the closing of the Intensive: "We commit to nurturing the script and growing it into what we feel is our story to tell."

Working through all these reactions can be facilitated when viewing the projections as a parallel process to recovery. CoATT assigns a dual task to CP and Participant here: to tolerate the fear, anger, and disappointment of the cast upon script reading. The newly recovered individual will encounter emotional challenges that must be worked through from the perspective of active recovery.

Movement Five: Rehearsal

During Rehearsal weeks, we stage and rehearse the play, and always return to the commitment and rehearsal concept to drive the work. If adjunct facilitators – such as interns or paraprofessionals – are part of the project, CP1 can be working on the play scene by scene while non-working group members are running lines, or working on character development. Additionally, participants may want individual support, such as to suggest rewrites to the script. We encourage this, with the caveat that any change to one character's lines will likely change the lines and scene for other characters. So, although we give every participant the right to rewrite lines until they are satisfied they have it right, they must gain the approval of the group to institute changes that might change the story at large. Theatre-makers will see how laborious and time-consuming this process may become, but it is essential that the participants are co-creating the material at every level. CoATT productions are built on the script, and the script is co-active. Additionally, the practice of voicing needs, mentalizing with other participants, and concretely making those changes is invaluable.

The need for co-active creation is one factor that differentiates CoATT rehearsal from traditional theatrical rehearsal. CP1 may be leading the process and may take the lead in staging the production. Given the therapeutic stance and focus on recovery, however, the movement flexes in duration to accommodate the capacity of the group, availability of space, and ability to master the material. It is common to add extra weeks in the Rehearsal movement, as it is often where people need the most support in relating the role to recovery and gaining the confidence to put on the performance.

The ensemble is as critical to supporting recovery as it is to delivering a performance, but the rehearsal phase is filled with individual challenges, struggles, availability, and levels of involvement. During the rehearsal phase, we have manualized a change to the session structure that promotes co-active facilitation of the process. A warm-up exercise must open the session, but the model asks a participant to take charge by choosing and leading this activity.

Closing exercises each week remain an important way to maintain the connection between participants. A participant facilitates the closing. Perhaps the individual leads the "Magic Pot" to close rehearsals: letting go of something you don't want to take with you and finding something you want to take away with you that can be attached to your body metaphorically. CP1 continues to support recovery through demonstrating the process of rehearsing a play and how that parallels independent recovery. Participants may begin to sponta-neously observe this connection and reinforce it for each other.

In this stage, the group may begin to shift into loving the play, their roles, and the message they have carefully crafted. Not only are participants taking in the messages from the roles they are playing and making connections between their role and their own recovery, but they are also adding the role of "artist" to their repertoire. The group usually begins to feel healthier in their active recovery, as well as supporting one another in group health. While this can be scary, using the playmaking process and supporting the group in relating the rehearsal process to recovery is essential, both on the stage and off.

We also note for the cast that the word Rehearsal contains the phrase "re-hear." The focus on re-hearing is the key to creating openness for successful rehearsal. Participants need openness to see others perform their lines, to try to understand and perform the lines in the script in different ways, and to be changed by playing the scenes. Most participants get stuck saying a line the same way or playing a scene the same way. In these moments, we come back to re-hearing. We ask them to go back to the theme that the group selected and to act in line with recovery and the metaphor that is being used. Re-hearing the theme of the play is extraordinarily useful for grounding parti-cipants and simultaneously strengthening recovery. We have found that static line readings and false performances happen when the participant has not figured out how to connect the moment in the performance to their recovery – the life-drama connection is missing. CoATT participants have an advantage over traditional actors because they know that the exploration is in service of recovery. When reminded of this tool they can explore a moment through this additional lens. When we re-hear the moment, connect it to our theme, and relate it to individual recovery, both metaphorically in the play and con-cretely to life, we bolster the play and recovery itself.

Remember, too, that the participants are getting ready to do a show. Rehearsal is continuing as usual while keeping the above in mind. Participants begin to work with the props that they will use in the production and begin to design costumes. This is an important step, as the costumes and props may become a transitional object kept after the event as a physical reminder of the relationships and the process. Here, paying close attention and using the clinical eye is important, as this shows up in small ways. For one client in eating disorder recovery who identified as Jewish Modern Orthodox – a belief system that has strict rules about women and modesty – it was about wearing a very specific pair of jeans, which signified both something about her recovery and her relationship to her Judaism as a woman. For another cast member, it was a tracksuit that he really wanted his character to wear, and that he himself wanted to wear proudly in his recovery.

During the Rehearsal movement, the group is also tasked with designing a co-active element to facilitate the audience during the production. The goal is an experience that will create a shared understanding between the cast and the community at large. We are looking for something beyond a talkback. We look to the theme of the play rather than reenrolling participants as the "sick one" and audience members as "the voyeuristic one." We work to level the power dynamic by designing an interactive element inviting the audience to participate in a healthy risk related to the theme of the play. The co-active audience element works to strengthen what Judith Herman calls "reconnection to community" (Herman, 2015).

It also empowers the participants to become directors. Here, they work together to design the element and execute it with the audience alongside CP1. Typically, the participants invite audience members to make, perform, or participate in an activity that results in a piece of art. Whether this is a poem, a book of photos, or breathing together at the end of the play, this last step is a concrete demonstration that individuals in recovery are a part of the community and can make a meaningful contribution that comes from their own experiences. The artifacts from these co-active experiences serve as concrete proof.

The many tasks of producing a public performance must be handled by CP1 with the support of the team and participants. For example, an audience must be invited with materials such as a poster or other social media elements. Some participants want to take on these elements as part of their process and should do so with the support of the group. If not, the group can discuss with CP1 the images or ideas that can be used for the poster and playbill.

Technical rehearsals of the play are like those for a typical theatrical run, focused on the operation of lights, sound, scenery, and props. If your CoATT production has the support of interns for these technical concerns, you may consider therapeutic approaches to that work (Smittle, 2017).

Gathering an audience is important for a CoATT production, as well as a typical theatre production. Preparing participants for the audience encounter is related to the recovery process in the most direct of ways, though. The audience encounter is the singular point of the CoATT model, as it represents the moment of stepping into the lowest levels of care, living in active recovery, and joining with the community as a newly recovered person. There are as many fears around inviting friends and family as there are around a public audience. Rather than trying to control, predict, and curate an audience, it is in service of recovery to prepare participants for any number of audience outcomes; it serves as a parallel to recovery. Individuals are responsible for their own recovery, but they cannot control the way others may respond to it.

Different populations may face different trigger points. Clients with eating disorders should be prepared for this well-meaning person who says, "you look so healthy!" Alternatively, clients with aphasia should be prepared for the audience member who focuses solely on the parts of the play where participants said the line "just perfect!" These interactions *will* happen in our participants' lives, and using this process as an opportunity to practice recovery-based responses is an empowering one.

We work to prepare participants for this eventuality via a discussion, role-play practice, or guided imagery. We bring awareness to the fear, support, and strategies needed to tolerate those feelings, such as imagining a positive outcome that is in the control of the participant. After the discussion, participants may also realize there was someone they were avoiding inviting for this very reason. If the participant feels settled and resolved about inviting that person, we encourage them to send an invitation.

Movement Six: Public Performance

In the CoATT Model, the theatre production must culminate in a performance that includes a public audience. The play provides an opportunity for participants to take risks, be vulnerable, and offer value to their communities. As mentioned, because there is no talkback experience with the audience, the play ends with a co-creation element designed and facilitated by the cast to help the audience reflect on the performance. In the same way that CPs and participants have been co-active in the process, the participants also become co-active with the audience in exploring their theme of recovery.

Each production comes with many feelings after the final bow and co-active elements take place. We strongly recommend, when possible, that the cast gather afterward for light refreshments and processing. It is a wonderful time for participants to take in the genuine experiences of the audience, which most often are awe, wonder, tenderness, joy, pride, and the like. It is also important with some populations, like eating disorders and substance use recovery, that there is state-based reality testing against the internal negative self-talk that can arise. Participants realize that, in fact, no one noticed that a line was forgotten, or that a prop was missing. More often, what many cast members realize is that it is hard to take in compliments and to be witnessed in a new role. When this happens, real-time reflection on life in active recovery is activated. This is excellent material to work through in everyday life: "How does it feel to encounter others and allow them to have an opinion about me?" As the participants move away from the CoATT process in the Launch phase, they will carry this awareness and skill into encounters in their community. They may not be in another play, but the same comments may arise at work, in the family setting, or in romantic pursuit. During the Launch movement, these post-show experiences are often processed just as much as the performance itself.

Movement Seven: Launch

In this final movement, the group will reflect upon the experience, solidify the relationships that have been built, and terminate the work of the CPs. These sessions should be scheduled before the Public Performance and should occur at least a week after the presentation. The name implies the action in this movement: Participants launch themselves into the community.

The Launch phase is crucial to the completion of the model and to the post-process experience of the participants. It is documented that after production, individuals may experience a bit of post-show depression, and general drama therapy treatment recommends there be ample space to process (Emunah & Johnson, 1983). CoATT goes one step further here, and requires not just meaning-making, but also concrete goal-setting. Although we make space for the transition and loss in ending the process, we also aim to highlight for participants the embodied nature of the work, and the way the body can be used as a meaningful tool in the world to make change. The body has been the location of the active recovery, as well as the vehicle for connecting to the community. Participants will want to plan to continue active recovery through goal setting.

We ask participants to think about something action-based that is measurable and achievable in order to utilize support, and even enhance their recovery. As group members share and process, we use the prompt: "What wisdom does the play, the character you played, or the rehearsal process have for you about your goal?" For example, participants who played artists have committed to obtaining art tools, and one participant who sang to the characters that were her children in the play committed to singing to her adult children in real life.

Together, we look at artifacts from the co-active audience element. In one production the co-active element asked the audience to write messages in a yearbook with their hopes for the future. In another production, the coactive element provided the audience with a two-sided mask and asked them to illustrate what is shown to the world and what is hidden. For each production the artifact will reflect the theme of the play, so participants collect a physical reminder of the experience. Looking at the audience artifacts is an enjoyable part of the process and helps solidify to participants that the work they intended to do made an impact on the audience in a meaningful way. The participants may choose to have some artifacts archived so that they remain available to be viewed. Readers may view some of our archives at https://www.recoverythroughperformance.org/past-productions-copy.

Finally, CP1 invites the participants to prepare for and attend a cast party. The group may want to organize a participant party (and for substance use disorder populations, distinctly naming that as a "sober party" is essential) to celebrate the relationships they have developed and their artistic achievement. This has had many forms depending on the population. Additionally, allowing the participants to plan the party they want is another confidence-boosting act for the group. They will be practicing what they learned in the play by celebrating in the community. Joyous events among friends, colleagues, and fellow travelers are a wonderful expression of active recovery.

Reference List

Emunah, R., & Johnson, D. R. (1983). The impact of theatrical performance on the self-images of psychiatric patients. *The Arts in Psychotherapy*, *10*(4): 233–239. 10.1016/0197-4556(83)90024-2

Guest, C. (1996). *Waiting for Guffman* [film]. Castle Rock Entertainment.

Herman, Judith. (2015). *Trauma and recovery*. Basic Books.

Landy, R. J. (1994). *Drama therapy: Concepts, theories and practices* (2nd ed.). Charles C. Thomas. https://psycnet.apa.org/record/1994-98841-000

Landy, R. J. (1996). *Persona and performance: The meaning of role in drama, therapy, and everyday life*. Guilford Press. https://psycnet.apa.org/record/1994-97043-000

Recovery Through Performance. (n.d.). *RTP archive*. https://www.recoverythroughperformance.org/past-productions-copy

Schwartz, R. C. (1995). *Internal family systems*. Guilford.

Schwartz, R. C., & Sweezy, M. (2019). *Internal family systems therapy* (2nd ed.). Guilford.

Smittle, E. (2017). *A guiding light: Establishing design within Therapeutic Theatre* [Unpublished master's thesis]. New York University.

Stevens, A. (2023). BART, The Black American Role Taxonomy: A Culturally Expansive Approach to Role Theory and Method Breathing Beyond Borders: Racial Justice and Decolonial Healing Practices. *Drama Therapy Review*, 9(1): 81–99.

Warphotography. (2009, July 11). *Ira Glass on storytelling 3* [YouTube]. Video. https://www.youtube.com/watch?v=X2wLP0izeJE

Wood, L. L. (2016). *The use of therapeutic theater in supporting clients in eating disorder recovery after intensive treatment: A qualitative study* [Doctoral dissertation, University of Missouri, St. Louis]. UMSL Libraries. https://irl.umsl.edu/dissertation/21

Wood, L. L., & Mowers, D. (2019). The Co-Active Therapeutic Theatre model: A manualized approach to creating therapeutic theatre with persons in recovery. *Drama Therapy Review*, 5(2): 217–234. 10.1386/dtr_00003_1

Chapter 4

The CoATT Model

A Step-by-Step Guide to Creating Therapeutic Theatre

This chapter presents the detailed manualization of the model. We do suggest that, before jumping into this chapter, readers are familiar with the previous chapters in order to understand the implications of manualization, as well as the operationalized terms that will appear in this chapter. As outlined in the introduction, to our knowledge, CoATT is the first manualized model of therapeutic theatre. Manualization is useful in that it provides a way of replicating the process, making it ideal for randomized control trials – a necessary step toward becoming an Evidence-Based Treatment/Practice (EBT/P).

Manualization requires three core components: 1) competence, which ensures that people are properly trained in the model and have the overall skill set, knowledge, and attitude in delivering the protocol; 2) adherence, which means the protocol is delivered as intended; and 3) fidelity, which is the tool used to ensure that competence and adherence are present in the delivery of the study (Cassiello-Robbins et al., 2022). When practitioners meet these three requirements, they are delivering a manualized CoATT production. If a production selects isolated ideas or exercises, delivers the model with only one CoATT Practitioner ("CP"), or makes other major modifications, it is a CoATT "inspired" production, and results would not qualify toward our efforts of creating an EBT/P. Again, we are thrilled with whatever way individuals want to use the model, as long as it meets the needs of your group.

EBTs have been criticized for being too rigid and for not allowing for the flexibility to respond to real client needs in the moment (Cassiello-Robbins et al., 2022). Regarding the notion of manualizing therapeutic theatre, we have encountered two primary concerns from fellow practitioners: 1) that manualization will suffocate flexibility, freedom, and spontaneity, and 2) the articulated difficulty of adherence to the model during the creative process. CoATT acknowledges these concerns and addresses them by offering a manualized model that offers flexibility by considering the client's worldview (e.g., active recovery, choosing a theme, being co-active) their capacity (e.g., multiple warm-up/closing options), and the duration, both in session length and number of weeks, that each movement is offered. Each CP must be

DOI: 10.4324/9781003161608-5

mindful in developing a responsible, critical, and theoretical appreciation of where their client's worldview and definition of recovery comes from through an appreciation of each individual's circumstance.

Regarding the concern about adherence during a creative process, we have developed the Movement Scorecard (MS) as a tool to aid you in research endeavors while applying the model. If you are not conducting research, it can be used to support treatment planning, or as a training tool while you are learning the model. If you are delivering a *CoATT-inspired* production, you may not need this tool.

We also want to be clear that we do not see manualization as the sole pathway toward creating change in the field. We are aware that maunalization is not yet prevalent in drama therapy or in applied theatre. However, drama therapists, counselors, and applied theatre artists work in spaces where the use of EBT/P holds power. Thus, our manual potentially empowers practitioners to advocate for client resources. Manualization has not necessarily proved to be a more effective form of treatment, but rather, is conducive to quantitative research (Truijens et al., 2019).

The model can, however, support practitioners in explaining the process to colleagues in an institutional setting, given that we use language and structures familiar to these settings. Thus, CoATT may also give drama therapists or other practitioners some leverage with a treatment team, grant-writing, and/or partnering with institutions that subscribe to a medical model.

We also acknowledge some of the expressed concerns about quantitative research. Historically, white college-aged men are a predominant sample, with results assumed to apply to other groups without regard to gender, ethnicity, or underrepresented groups. Thus, every CoATT pilot study with a new population includes qualitative research to support the discovery of what participants identify as being beneficial. We then use those results to inform our selection of valid and reliable quantitative measures for future productions. This allows us to avoid a common pitfall of quantitative research, in that the scales we pick are rooted in results derived from participants' input (Truijens et al., 2019). Additionally, many of the groups we work with, especially BIPOC individuals or those with psychiatric disorders, may be suspicious of research, given the complex history of unethical research on vulnerable populations (Brandt, 1978; Fulford &Howse, 1993). Thus, beyond a sound Institutional Review Board approval, we have open conversations about the aims of our research. We acknowledge the historically harmful past, as well as make space to hear narratives about personal research experiences that have been ethical but have made participants feel like "specimens." We share our goal to create an evidence-based treatment that is based in the arts, community, and participant experience. When we are radically transparent about why we do research, create a culture of inquiry about our research alongside reminding participants about their explicit right to not do the research component and still be in the production, we find great enthusiasm and individuals who express the transformative experience of having research be presented with authenticity and transparency.

For those of you who are conducting research with the model at the pilot level, we have also included our most used version of our qualitative protocol (Appendix E).

Beyond participant experiences, we have also measured caregiver, provider, or audience responses, and researchers using the model can consider the same. We support arts-based research approaches in tandem with quantitative research. Arts-based processes can enhance understanding of the ephemeral qualities that can be hard to capture in quantitative research (Leavy, 2017).

We offer these suggestions and modifications to address these larger systemic issues that arise around quantitative research and EBT/P's. We strive toward the creation of an EBT/P that is both sound in its manualization for research purposes and addresses long-neglected feedback from research participants (Drisko & Grady, 2019). We aim for research, like the model, to be driven by curiosity and co-action (Drisko & Grady, 2019).

Specific Tasks in the CoATT Model

The CoATT model is made up of seven movements that can happen over the course of 10–16 weeks, or more. The number of weeks can be adjusted based on how often you are able to meet with participants and the constraints of the organization you are partnering with, as well as stipulations from funding or treatment protocols. We do not recommend more than a 20-week process, though, in order to ensure the participants are able to launch and transition into the next stage of their recovery. The priority and success of the model mainly rely on the delivery of the seven movements in sequential order, as well as a CoATT team that understands their recovery population.

A movement in the model can be understood as a movement in classical music. Each movement in CoATT has its own feel, sound, and rhythm, and propels the piece at large. In CoATT, there are seven movements, and each movement is made up of five notes. The five notes are important as they create clear anticipatory guidance for all involved in the project. Most movements call for multiple phases (e.g., Movement Two, Phase One) to allow for the completion of important tasks in the group process and the development of the theme. Typically, one session is dedicated to each phase. Based on group needs, CPs may spend more than one session per phase. Fidelity to the CoATT Model does not require a specific duration, but it does require that all tasks are completed (Figure 4.1).

The **participant task** is the expectation of what the performers in the play will be physically or emotionally doing and exploring in each session, and is written in action-based language.

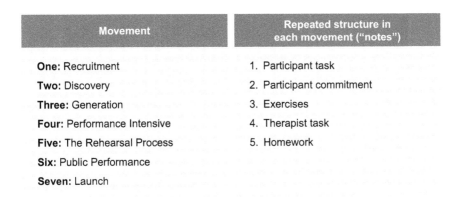

Movement	Repeated structure in each movement ("notes")
One: Recruitment	1. Participant task
Two: Discovery	2. Participant commitment
Three: Generation	3. Exercises
Four: Performance Intensive	4. Therapist task
Five: The Rehearsal Process	5. Homework
Six: Public Performance	
Seven: Launch	

Figure 4.1 The Seven Movements and Five Notes of CoATT.

The **participant commitment** is a mechanism to enroll each participant in the work of each session, supporting a co-active working relationship. It describes the emotional investment that each participant makes in the process. This is essential in working with folks in recovery as it is a way for them to have clear expectations and practice taking self-responsibility, and is a way for the group to have a system of confronting or challenging individuals in the group process.

The participant task and participant commitment are essential tools we use to track the process. They are also used as a grounding factor for participants and for the treatment centers we partner with. Many participants or partnering treatment centers have no context for putting on a production; they are excited about the idea of it but knowing how it comes together and trusting that process can be very difficult. Each week, we ensure that this task and commitment are clear and known. When a participant feels anxious, worried, or lost (oftentimes, these are old patterns related to their recovery being projected onto the CoATT process), bringing them back to the weekly task and commitment provides context and anchoring. For treatment center staff who work with the clients throughout the week, or for individual therapists who may inquire about what their client is working on, the participant task and commitment give clear, actionable language to help support their clients. It also provides language that can be included on treatment plans or for insurance purposes, when required. Participants are absolutely welcome to take the spirit of the commitment and put it into their own words. The words here serve as a starting point.

There is a sense of ritual attached to the participant commitment, which is underlined by the way it is positioned in each session of the model. Like all rituals, reciting the participant commitment helps to mark progress through a process. Each community adapts ritual practices to create deeper meaning and access for the individuals participating. Consider any academic calendar in which Back to School and Graduation are established rituals; the events themselves may look very different at different institutions. CPs co-actively adapt the presentation of the weekly participant commitment to create meaning for their group. Some groups may recite the commitment as a pledge, others may dedicate a certain amount of time for discussion, still others may make a visual presentation to keep the commitment alive in the rehearsal room, and others may create a physical sculpture representing the commitment.

The **exercises** are specifically designed and scaffolded and are facilitated by the CPs. They have been sequenced to take participants on a journey, to generate material, to create aesthetic distance, to strengthen recovery, and to move the group toward a final public production. Each exercise sequence is broken into three parts. First, there is the warm-up, which includes going over the participant commitment, as well as a dramatic exercise that prepares the individuals' mind and body for the work of the day. Next is the core, which are the exercises that take up the bulk of time in the session and are used to support discovering a theme, generating material, building cohesion, and strengthening recovery. Finally, there is a closing in which participants have an opportunity to reflect on the dramatic work, relate it to recovery, and re-regulate their bodies and emotions.

The **therapist task** provides a clear checklist to hold the facilitator(s) accountable for the emotional and physical work that is taking place with participants. This also helps define the difference in roles between participant and CP and ensures that the material between sessions is being used to move the work toward production. The therapist's task also denotes which co-leader will be facilitating.

Finally, **the homework** is the work that will be done between sessions by the participants. The homework is used to strengthen the group work, generate material for the play, create a container for the thoughts and ideas of the participants, help the participants connect beyond the rehearsal space, and act as an informal assessment tool to understand the progress of the participants. The homework should be kept organized in a designated space, as it is instrumental to script writing. We usually have an intern, or person who is part of the sponsoring organization, collect and organize homework each week. Homework can also be stored on a password-protected Google Doc so that the participants can read each other's work. If qualitative research is being conducted, homework can serve as another data point in the research process, with proper Institutional Review Board (IRB) approval. One consideration to keep in mind is that some populations may do better with homework being woven into session time. For example, we found that for participants with schizophrenia, the homework was deterring them from participation. We found that we were able to meet the group "where they were" by working elements of the homework into the sessions. We have delineated home assignments for each movement in the manual.

Reading the Manual

As you read through the manual, you will see that many of our directions are written plainly. In fact, we often use the language "Say: XYZ," though we do not mean that you literally need to dictate these instructions word for word. We are trying to provide a sense of a script for you to best explain the exercises. You may decide that the group needs more warm-up time, and you may add on additional theatre games, or other changes. This is fine, but keep in mind that, for research purposes, you will need to note modifications made in your limitations section.

We had the pleasure of working with a group of students at Lesley University, in Boston, MA, in the summer of 2022. They were tasked with reading an exercise from the manual and executing it on the spot with a group of students enrolled as participants. First-, second-, and third-year students were able to read the exercises and execute them properly. This group also provided essential wording tips to maximize clarity and effectiveness.

Movement One: Recruitment and Screening

Duration: Flexible. This process can take as many weeks as desired by the CoATT team and, if relevant, partnering organization. If research is being conducted, all necessary approvals should be acquired before the start of the recruitment process. If research is not being conducted, pre-project team meetings, designation of dates of the project, and various role designations and relationships between the CoATT team and partnering facilities should take place.

Who: Both CP1 and CP2 are involved in Movement One.

CP Task: A clear, structured recruitment and screening process is central to CoATT and its success. The sponsoring organization should offer a general information session as a primary recruiting tool. This general information session should describe the project and its parameters, and the time commitment, and culminating public performance must be made clear. Equally important, all candidates must be clear that this is a therapeutic intervention timed to support them in their recovery. Successful screening relies on a strong clinical understanding of the population that will be working on the production. Keep in mind the cognitive ability, physical limitations, emotional maturity and stability, and demographic makeup of the group.

Movement Scorecard (MS) for CoATT

General Instructions

The team should decide who will score the MS based on the research design. If no research is taking place, the MS can be omitted or scored by CP1. Options include the individual delivering the intervention and/or an outside rater trained in CoATT. If the MS is being filled out by the individual delivering the intervention, the MS should be filled out directly after session for fidelity purposes. If a task scores less than a 2, it should be denoted and described in the protocol notes section at the end of the MS.

The following scale should be used to rate the degree to which the warm-up was completed by circling the number.

0 ······· Concept/exercise was not delivered by the practitioner

1 ······· Concept/exercise was partially delivered by the practitioner

2 ······· Concept/exercise was fully delivered by the practitioner

Movement	Recruitment
Duration	Flexible
Facilitated by	CP1 and 2, Partnering Organization
Session Length	N/A
Overview	Participants are recruited, screened, and prepared for the process
Participant Task	The participant task in movement one is to answer the recruitment questions as dictated by the co-active team, with a specific emphasis on active recovery
Participant Commitment	"I have committed to this project and am trying something new in service of my recovery."
Practitioner Task	Deliver a thoughtful recruitment and screening process based on clinical expertise*
Homework	1. CoATT Strengths and Resources Form (Appendix F) 2. CoATT Relapse Prevention Plan (if applicable) 3. Any paperwork as required by the research team

Date: _____

PRACTITIONER TASKS

Recruitment	0	1	2
Screening	0	1	2
Forms collected	0	1	2
Calendar provided	0	1	2

WARM-UP

N/A	0	1	2
	0	1	2
	0	1	2

CORE

N/A	0	1	2

CLOSING

N/A	0	1	2
	0	1	2

Homework given: ☐ Yes   ☐ No

Notes for manualization exercises not fully executed:

CoATT Practitioner: _____

MS completed by: _____

Role to project: _____

Figure 4.2 **Movement One scorecard for CoATT.**

Note: If partnering with another organization, consider using a pre-process partnership checklist. See Appendix A.

Screening and recruitment can happen over the phone, via email, through a questionnaire, an in-person paper application, or some combination of these options. For research purposes, this will be standardized based on the design of the study. For some populations, you may require a letter of approval from the individual's primary therapist or psychiatrist to ensure treatment coordination and readiness. Those spearheading recruitment and screening should have a way of clearly delivering and documenting their process. For a research process, a standardized approach should be agreed to and followed for all applications to the process. And, for purposes of equity, the standardized screening process must be made explicit.

Participant task: The participant task in movement one is to answer the recruitment questions as dictated by the co-active team, with a specific emphasis on active recovery. These questions will reflect the subject matter expertise of the treatment team.

Participant commitment: "I have committed to this project and am trying something new in service of my recovery."

Homework: Once participants are accepted to be a part of the project, they are asked to fill out the following: 1) CoATT Strengths and Resources Form (Appendix F) 2) CoATT Relapse Prevention Plan (if applicable) 3) Any paperwork as required by the research team (Figure 4.2).

Movement Two: Discovery[1]

Movement Two, Phase One

Duration: Flexible. Typically, a two-hour group meets once a week for two weeks. However, the capacity of participants should be taken into consideration.

Who: CP1

Overview: Participants apply dramatic exploration to the concept of embodied recovery to identify potential themes of the play.

Commitment: "This show is about working in service of our active recovery the entire time."

Participant Task: Participants focus on telling their recovery story by embodying and embracing recovery.

CP Task: CP1 reviews the participant's commitment with the group. CP1 reminds the group that the goal of the session is to answer the CoATT question: "What is a theme of recovery you want to create a play in service of strengthening your recovery and sharing with an audience?" CP1 delivers the appropriate warm-up, core, and closing based on group needs and manualized exercises. This is the only session that has an autobiographical focus before the production moves away from a personal narrative and embraces group metaphor.

Exercises

Warm-up (choose one based on group capacity)

- *Sound and Movement:* The session begins with participants coming into a circle and introducing themselves. During the second time around, they introduce themselves with a sound and a movement about how they are feeling about beginning the CoATT process. The group discusses how we could learn something about someone else just through sound and movement. We use this to teach the group that we can express a great deal with more than just words, and that this concept will be key to our production.
- *Warm-up Walks:* The group is asked to move around the room slowly, as if honey is on the floor, and then quickly, as if they are being chased by bees. They are asked to move in the space as if there was a rain cloud in their body, and as if filled by a glowing light. We impart that by embodying different ways of being; we can experience those ways of feeling more acutely.

Core

- *Embody your Recovery:* Tie the above warm-up to the core exercise: "Just as we have embodied different ways of feeling/being in the space, we now invite the group to move in the space as if you are embodying your recovery as it is today." When embodied, recovery becomes Recovery, a character. Recovery is asked to move as if Recovery is tired, as if Recovery is motivated, or like any other characteristics of Recovery that can be named. Next, ask the participants to freeze their bodies in a static sculpt that expresses something about Recovery, as if they were sculptures in a museum. Say, "just looking at the sculpture we could learn something about one's recovery. Now I am going to give you a script. The first script is 'My name is Recovery and what I want more than anything is____.'" CP1 taps each participant and prompts the same line. Then, repeat with the following scripts: "My name is Recovery and what is blocking me is____." "My name is Recovery and something or someone that can help me is ____."
- Once all participants have enacted these three questions, a chair is placed in the middle of the room, and the rest of the chairs are set up audience style. Each person is invited to embody Recovery and give a one-minute monologue in the role of Recovery. The participants watching are enrolled as "compassionate/curious witnesses," and after the monologue are invited to ask the participant in the role of Recovery any clarifying questions. Participants can begin the monolouge with the script above, if they wish. They should speak from the role of Recovery. After each monologue allow the person to "de-role" and join the witnesses.
- Once each person has improvised their monologue, CP1 asks the group to list some shared themes they heard from the monologues. CP1 directs the group

Movement Scorecard (MS) for CoATT

General Instructions

The team should decide who will score the MS based on the research design. Options include the individual delivering the intervention and/or an outside rater trained in CoATT. If the MS is being filled out by the individual delivering the intervention, the MS should be filled out directly after session for fidelity purposes. If a task scores less than a 2, it should be denoted and described in the protocol notes section at the end of the MS.

The following scale should be used to rate the degree to which the warm-up was completed by circling the number.

0 ······ Concept/exercise was not delivered by
the practitioner

1 ······ Concept/exercise was partially delivered by
the practitioner

2 ······ Concept/exercise was fully delivered by
the practitioner

Movement	Discovery
Duration	Flexible
Facilitated by	CP1
Session Length	2 hours
Overview	Participants apply dramatic exploration to the concept of embodied recovery to identify potential themes of the play.
Participant Task	Participants focus on telling their recovery story by embodying and embracing recovery.
Participant Commitment	"This show is about working in service of our active recovery the entire time."
Practitioner Task	Lead group toward thematic answers to the CoATT question
Homework	Participants will journal and submit to the CoATT team "What do you want from recovery and what is blocking you?"

Date: _____

WARM-UP

Share participant commitment	0	1	2
Discuss the CoATT Question	0	1	2
Deliver one of two warm-ups	0	1	2

CORE

Embody recovery	0	1	2
Identify shared themes of recovery	0	1	2

CLOSING

Moving body to re-regulate	0	1	2
Link themes to recovery question	0	1	2

Homework given: ☐ Yes   ☐ No

Notes for manualization exercises not fully executed:

CoATT Practitioner: _____

MS completed by: _____

Role to project: _____

Figure 4.3 Movement Two, Phase One scorecard for CoATT.

to create a new sculpture expressing the shared themes: the group builds a fluid sculpt of that theme and offers a line, sound, and movement. When CP1 points to different participants, they repeat the line, sound, or movement, creating a Greek chorus. CP1 points in different patterns to highlight various narratives of the theme. Perform as many themes as time permits.

Closing

- *Magic Pot:* The group comes together in the circle again and shakes off the different parts of their body, using this to re-regulate themselves from the exploration. Say, "In the circle there is a pot, it holds both something you want to leave behind from the first session, and something you want to take with you." Direct participants to physically take something out of their body to leave behind, and to fill up their body with something new from the group that they physically place in their body to take with them.

Homework: Participants will journal in whatever format is suitable to them and submit to the CoATT team an answer to the question: "What do you want from recovery and what is blocking you?" (Figure 4.3)

Movement Two, Phase Two

Duration: 2–4 sessions

Who: CP1

Overview: Participants use future projection in service of clarifying the message for their play.

Participant Commitment: "We commit to working towards a meaningful theme that will benefit our recovery and the community at large."

Participant Task: Participants are working through metaphor to solidify a theme that is in service of strengthening recovery. This will then drive the show and character choices, and heighten the meaning-making in the play creation process.

CP Task: Introduce the participant's commitment. Highlight common themes that are coming up in the group in the exercises and homework. Deliver the warm-up, core, and closing.

Exercises

Warm-up (choose one based on group capacity)

- *Sound and Movement:* The session begins with participants coming into a circle and introducing themselves. During the second time going around, they introduce themselves with a sound and movement with how they are feeling this week in recovery.
- *Postcard from the future:* The group stands in a circle. CP1 says, "Show me a sculpt about how you are feeling today in recovery. When I tap you, change the sculpt to show me what you will feel like five years from now. Once you have changed the sculpt, I will tap you on the shoulder and give you the script. "I am the future of recovery, the biggest things that are different about me are_____"

Movement Scorecard (MS) for CoATT

General Instructions

The team should decide who will score the MS based on the research design. Options include the individual delivering the intervention and/or an outside rater trained in CoATT. If the MS is being filled out by the individual delivering the intervention, the MS should be filled out directly after session for fidelity purposes. If a task scores less than a 2, it should be denoted and described in the protocol notes section at the end of the MS.

The following scale should be used to rate the degree to which the warm-up was completed by circling the number.

0 ······ Concept/exercise was not delivered by the practitioner

1 ······ Concept/exercise was partially delivered by the practitioner

2 ······ Concept/exercise was fully delivered by the practitioner

Movement	Discovery
Duration	2–4 sessions
Facilitated by	CP1
Session Length	2 hours
Overview	Participants use future projection in service of clarifying the message for their play
Participant Task	Participants are working through metaphor to solidify a theme that is in service of strengthening recovery which will drive the show, character choices, and heighten the meaning making in the play process.
Participant Commitment	"We commit to working towards a meaningful theme that will benefit our recovery and the community at large."
Practitioner Task	Encouraging the group to test their themes of the play against active recovery
Homework	Journal about two themes that the group is thinking about exploring and how they relate to your own personal recovery.

Date: _____

WARM-UP

Share participant commitment	0	1	2
Deliver one of two warm ups	0	1	2

CORE

Future talk show	0	1	2
Clarify common themes			
Compare working themes to group definition of active recovery			

CLOSING

Deliver one of two closing exercises	0	1	2

Homework given: ☐ Yes   ☐ No

Notes for manualization exercises not fully executed:

CoATT Practitioner: _____

MS completed by: _____

Role to project: _____

Figure 4.4 Movement Two, Phase Two scorecard for CoATT.

Core

- *Future Talk Show:* In the future talk show, CP1 and the group will interview each member as the character they just created from the warm-up: a version of themselves in recovery five years from now. Enroll all participants as talk show audience members until it is their turn to be interviewed.. Each participant will get at least one question from CP1, who is the host, and may also take questions from the audience. Questions should be open-ended and explore common themes in the group experience of recovery. Questions may also engage in fantasy or wish fulfillment.

  Transition out of the core exercise by de-roling our future selves through words or physical action.
- *Commit to Theme:* Together, the group then commits to a theme they want to explore through the play; the theme should be congruent with their initial definition of active recovery. At this point, there may be two or three themes, but the group is narrowing them down in preparation to begin further exploration next week.

Closing (choose one based on group capacity)

- *Magic Pot:* The group comes together in the circle again and shakes off the different parts of their body, using this to re-regulate from the exploration. Say, "In the circle there is a pot, it holds both something you want to leave behind from the first session, and something you want to take with you." Direct participants to physically take something out of their body to leave behind, and to fill up their body with something new from the group that they physically place in their body to take with them.
- *Future Feelings:* Stand in a circle and imagine a future audience has just watched you perform a play about one of these themes. Say, "I just performed a play for an audience about recovery. The audience felt _____ while watching it and I felt _____after performing it."

Homework: Journal about two themes that the group is thinking about exploring and how they relate to your own personal recovery (Figure 4.4).

Movement Three: Generation

Movement Three, Phase One

Duration: 3–5 sessions

Who: CP1

Overview: Participants use metaphor to explore and generate material in service of building a script.

Participant Commitment: "We commit to exploring the selected theme through role, story, and metaphor as related to the group and ourselves, in service of recovery."

Participant Task: Improvise and refine characters, relationships, and situations related to the theme of the play.

CP Task: Introduce the participant commitment. CP1 provides prompts and suggestions for dramatic exploration by emphasizing the theme, what we want an audience to know, and how what we are doing is related to recovery. Assign scenes and roles that support each person's developing role system. Collect scenes or monologues pertinent to each person's recovery. Catalog the material for use in movement four.

Exercises

Warm-up (choose one based on group capacity)

- *Sound and Movement:* The session begins with participants coming into a circle and introducing themselves. During the second time around, they introduce themselves with a sound and movement that reflects how they are feeling this week in recovery.
- *Zip, Zap Zop:* Standing in a circle, participants "pass" a connection through three different gestures: a) A first participant says: "zip" as they clap in the direction of another participant; b) The participant who receives the "zip" must say "zap" as they clap in the direction of another participant; c) The third participant must say "zop" as they pass to another participant. The cycle repeats or starts over if broken or incorrectly spoken. There are many editions and variations of this warm-up, and you are welcome to play your version if it facilitates focus, connection, listening, and spontaneity.

Core

- *Creating Characters:* CP1 provides a list of characters or generates a list of characters with participants.

  - Once the list is created or provided, participants select a character and begin by moving through the space as this character. Say, "How does this character walk with its feet, legs, torso, arms, head?" Allow participants to fully explore how a character moves in space. Then say, "Now greet someone in the space as this character." After they have met different characters in the space, have them shake off the character.
  - Say: "Now, we are going to do the same thing, but I will assign you a character." Lead the group through the same exploration as above.
  - Say: "Choose one of the two characters or a new character that you would like to explore more in-depth."

Movement Scorecard (MS) for CoATT

General Instructions

The team should decide who will score the MS based on the research design. Options include the individual delivering the intervention and/or an outside rater trained in CoATT. If the MS is being filled out by the individual delivering the intervention, the MS should be filled out directly after session for fidelity purposes. If a task scores less than a 2, it should be denoted and described in the protocol notes section at the end of the MS.

The following scale should be used to rate the degree to which the warm-up was completed by circling the number.

0 ······· Concept/exercise was not delivered by the practitioner

1 ······· Concept/exercise was partially delivered by the practitioner

2 ······· Concept/exercise was fully delivered by the practitioner

Movement	Generation
Duration	3–5 sessions
Facilitated by	CP1
Session Length	2 hours
Overview	Participants use metaphor to explore and generate material in service of building a script.
Participant Task	Improvise and refine characters, relationships, and situations related to the theme of the play
Participant Commitment	"We commit to exploring the selected theme through role, story, and metaphor as related to the group and ourselves, in service of recovery."
Practitioner Task	Inspiring and supporting spontaneous creation of dramatic material
Homework	Write two contrasting monologues from the characters and be prepared to share them or work with them next week.

Date: _____

WARM-UP

Share participant commitment	0	1	2
Deliver one of two warm ups	0	1	2
	0	1	2

CORE

Each participant creates two characters	0	1	2
Each participant performs one brief monologue	0	1	2
Reflect on characters created			

CLOSING

Deliver one of two closing exercises	0	1	2
	0	1	2

Homework given: ☐ Yes   ☐ No

Notes for manualization exercises not fully executed:

CoATT Practitioner: _____

MS completed by: _____

Role to project: _____

Figure 4.5 Movement Three, Phase One scorecard for CoATT.

- A chair is placed in the middle of the room and the rest of the chairs are set up audience style. Each person is invited to perform a short monologue from the character. The audience may ask questions to learn more about the character. At the end, de-role.
- CP1 asks, "What makes characters memorable, and which characters could be connected to the play we are imagining?"

Closing (choose one based on group capacity)

- *Magic Pot:* The group comes together in the circle again and shakes off the different parts of their body, using this to re-regulate from the exploration. Say, "In the circle there is a pot, it holds both something you want to leave behind from the first session, and something you want to take with you." Direct participants to physically take something out of their body to leave behind, and to fill up their body with something new from the group that they physically place in their body to take with them.
- *My Acting Resume:* The group comes together in the circle again and shakes off the different parts of their body, using this to re-regulate from the exploration. Say, "One way I am like the character I played today is_____. One way I am different from the character I played is_____."

Homework: Write two contrasting monologues from the characters and be prepared to share them, or work with them next week (Figure 4.5).

Movement Three, Phase Two

Duration: 4–6 sessions

Who: CP1 & CP2

Overview: Participants use metaphor to explore and generate material in service of building a script.

Participant Commitment: "We commit to exploring the selected theme through role, story, and metaphor as related to the group and ourselves, in service of recovery."

Participant Task: Improvise and refine characters, relationships, and situations as related to the theme of the play.

CP Task: CP1 prepares a list of appropriate scenes in consultation with CP2. The list should include situations and relationships for the characters who were presented in earlier sessions and may include new characters or situations that are relevant to the theme. CP1 must allow participants to develop the scenes without dictating content. CP1 teaches basic scene structure as having a beginning, a middle, and an end.

Exercises

Warm-up (choose one based on group capacity)

- *Sound and Movement:* The session begins with participants coming into a circle and introducing themselves. During the second time going around, they introduce themselves with a sound and movement reflecting how they are feeling this week in recovery.

Movement Scorecard (MS) for CoATT

General Instructions

The team should decide who will score the MS based on the research design. Options include the individual delivering the intervention and/or an outside rater trained in CoATT. If the MS is being filled out by the individual delivering the intervention, the MS should be filled out directly after session for fidelity purposes. If a task scores less than a 2, it should be denoted and described in the protocol notes section at the end of the MS.

The following scale should be used to rate the degree to which the warm-up was completed by circling the number.

0 ······· Concept/exercise was not delivered by
         the practitioner

1 ······· Concept/exercise was partially delivered by
         the practitioner

2 ······· Concept/exercise was fully delivered by
         the practitioner

Movement	Generation
Duration	4–6 sessions
Facilitated by	CP1
Session Length	2 hours
Overview	Participants use metaphor to explore and generate material in service of building a script.
Participant Task	Improvise and refine characters, relationships, and situations related to the theme of the play.
Participant Commitment	"We commit to exploring the selected theme through role, story, and metaphor as related to the group and ourselves, in service of recovery."
Practitioner Task	Generate and direct ten short scenes using characters created from previous session. Prepare participants for Intensive.
Homework	Write a scene using any two characters you witnessed during the week.

Date: _____

WARM-UP

Share participant commitment	0	1	2
Deliver one of two warm ups	0	1	2
	0	1	2

CORE

Facilitate improvisation of at least 5 scenes	0	1	2
Include every participant in at least one scene	0	1	2

CLOSING

Deliver one of two closing exercises	0	1	2
Discuss expectations for the Intensive	0	1	2

Homework given: ☐ Yes   ☐ No

Notes for manualization exercises not fully executed:

CoATT Practitioner: _____

MS completed by: _____

Role to project: _____

Figure 4.6. Movement Three, Phase Two scorecard for CoATT.

- *Mirroring:* Four rounds are offered, with participants finding a new partner each time: a) In the first round, participants find a partner and they mirror each other's body movements only; b) they then mirror each other's facial expressions; c) they mirror each other's voice; and d) they mirror all of the above. Reflect on the need to listen and watch one another when working on a scene.

Core

- Working from the list, improvised scenes are assigned between different characters, and participants play with the themes designated by the group. The group begins to focus on the structure of a scene: beginning, middle, and end.
- Prepare the group for the Intensive by discussing: What scenes did you enjoy? How do these scenes parallel recovery or the themes we are working on? Which scenes might you want to share with CP2?

Closing (choose one based on group capacity)

- *Magic Pot:* The group comes together in the circle again and shakes off the different parts of their body, using this to re-regulate from the exploration. Say, "In the circle there is a pot, it holds both something you want to leave behind from the first session, and something you want to take with you." Direct participants to physically take something out of their body to leave behind, and to fill up their body with something new from the group that they physically place in their body to take with them.
- *My Acting Resume:* The group comes together in the circle again and shakes off the different parts of their body, using this to re-regulate from the exploration. Say, "One way I am like the character I played today is_____. One way I am different from the character I played is_____."

Homework: Write a scene using any two characters you witnessed during the session. These may be explored in the next sessions during the Core in addition to repeating the protocol above (Figure 4.6).

Movement Four: Intensive

In the Intensive Movement, the different phases are denoted alphabetically rather than numerically. The notation is intended to indicate that CP2 leads these sessions and is working with the group to complete these tasks. It may also aid in organizing field notes for research purposes.

Duration: Three continuous sessions ("Intensive A," "B," and "C")

Intensive A

Who: CP2

Overview: Extended time for collaboration and creation of a first draft for production, which culminates in a reading of the script. Note: there are three sessions of work outlined. Sessions 6a and 6b may be collapsed in service of the needs and limitations of a particular population. Session 6c, the reading of the play, must always occur.

Participant Commitment: "We commit to working as part of an acting ensemble in collaboration with our co-active team."

Participant Task: Learn theatre skills in service of the production

Practitioner Task: Assessment of group readiness, inspire confidence, and develop resilience through teaching theatre skills

Exercises

Warm-up

- *Professional Introduction:* CP1 introduces CP2 as a theatre maker and partner for the group. CP2 introduces the concept of a specific set of skills for making a play. Participants introduce themselves and share their strengths in relation to the production. Participants may list characters they have played in the process so as to build on the previous closing exercise, "Acting Resume." Share participant commitment.

Core

Testing for Theatre Terminology: Choose one to three exercises to establish familiarity with rehearsal techniques and staging techniques.

- *Backup Line:* Ask participants to form a line across the back wall of the stage space. Ask participants to "walk downstage as a group." Ask participants to "show your back to the audience." Ask participants to "sit in the audience," then ask them to "return to the backup line in a different position." Teach "stage right" and "stage left" by directing participants one at a time to take a position. Direct participants to "exit stage right" and "exit stage left," as well as "enter stage right" and "enter stage left." Ask for a volunteer to play director and allow 3–5 participants to "give directions to the group."
- *Stage Picture:* Say something like, "Acting is easy because we just have to talk to each other and say our lines as truthfully as we can. But it's harder for an audience to follow a story, so we create a stage picture that they can understand just by looking." Put half the participants in the backup line and half in the audience. Say, "One at a time, walk downstage and take a frozen position like a statue. When you are frozen, the next person will walk downstage and make another statue, but the trick is that the second statue must be in a relationship with the first. Then, we will add on one at a time until we have a picture." When the stage picture is complete, ask one person in the audience to give a title to the picture. Ask one person in the picture to say what they think is happening in the picture.

- *Imaginary Environment:* Say, "We haven't even made up our play yet, but we are trying to imagine what the world of the play will be like. So, now we are going to create an imaginary space. In a moment, we will choose a type of environment. It will have one way IN and one way OUT. One at a time, everyone will come IN that way and go OUT that way. While you are IN, act like you are in the space. When you are OUT, change back to yourself." Ask the group what kind of environment they want to explore. Direct each participant one at a time as they enter and exit the space.
- *Imaginary Set:* Build on the Imaginary Environment by creating a specific location. Say, "This time we are going to make a specific place with many things inside it. This time, everyone will go IN and go OUT in the same spot. The first person, though, will add something into the space, like a window, a cabinet, a shelf, or refrigerator, or anything. They will show us that thing by interacting with it, and leave. The trick is that the second person will use the same object the first person did, and then add one more thing before she leaves. The third person will enter, use thing one and thing two, and add another one.
- *Moving Together:* Place groups of two to four participants in an imaginary vehicle. Using movement and sound, they should show us the vehicle in motion. Say, "Since you are all together, we want to see what it is like to be in this vehicle and how it moves you. When I say go, show us the vehicle in motion." Participants may suggest vehicles.

Creating Spontaneous Material with a New Member in the Room: Participants have grown comfortable making material with each other and with CP1, but CP2 is a new presence. CP2 may have been "built up" as a theatre expert, and the session may feel pressured because it has been called the "Intensive." Choose three to five exercises that encourage participants to improvise freely, and to make new material with CP2 watching and coaching.

- *18 Entrance Lines:* Ask half the group to create a backup line and half to be an audience. One at a time, participants leave the line and enter into a scene to say the opening line. When they have said a line, CP2 says "good" and they return to the back. This continues until the group has generated 18 entrance lines. Say, "We are going to make a script together this weekend, and we don't know where it will start, but it has to start somewhere. We already looked at locations and environments, now we will look at lines that might come up. I have a theory that location isn't the most important thing, because you can have many different scenes that happen in the same room. So, in a moment we will give the group a location. One at a time, you will walk into that location and say the FIRST line of a scene in that location. You can say ANY line that would start a scene in THAT location." Participants continue until 18 lines have been spoken. Rotate participants.

- *Describe the Box:* Place an imaginary box in the center of a circle. Ask the participants to describe the box. Each person adds one observable fact to the description of the box. Open the box and repeat the description of what the group finds inside. This exercise may be done in pairs. If so, ask the teams to share with the whole group what the box was like and what was inside.
- *Group Story, or What Happened Then?:* In a circle, each participant will say one sentence of a story at a time. After each sentence, CP2 (and often the whole group) will say "What happened then?" When the story resolves, CP2 leads the group in saying "The End."
- *Postcards:* Repeat the "Stage Pictures" exercise. This time, ask one participant to be the Author of the postcard. She will stand outside the group with her back to the stage. Ask three or five participants to be onstage. Say, "In a moment I will ask the people on stage to make a stage picture. They have fifteen seconds. When the fifteen seconds are up, I will say "freeze." The Author of the postcard will not see the picture until I say, "Take a look." After 15 seconds, CP2 will ask the 'author" to write a postcard message that would go with the picture. Before the onstage participants make the picture, ask the Author, "Who will you send the postcard to?" When everyone is ready, say "Go." Then "freeze." Ask the Author to turn and look at the picture. Ask her to start the postcard message with "Dear _____." The message should be three sentences long, and end with a closing salutation like, "Your son," "Sincerely," or "Very Truly Yours."
- *Instant Scene, or "Always Say the Next Logical Thing":* Participants create scenes through improvisation. Give each participant a 3 × 5 card and a pen. Ask them to finish the sentence, "I just saw _____" and write the whole sentence on the card. Place all the cards in a hat. Invite the participants to stand in the backup line. One person will take the card. That person will enter SECOND. They will join the participant who has entered FIRST and has started doing something in the space. Say, "Well, we're getting really good at imagining all the parts of the play. And I know you have been working on scenes together. Let's start a scene this way: One person will enter and start doing something in the location, so we know what it is. The person with the card will enter and say the line on the card. Then, we will get a reaction from the first person. See how many lines we can add on, taking turns. All you need to know is "say the next logical thing."
- *Instant Character:* Participants sit in a chair and make huge, weird, funny faces until CP2 says "freeze." Participants create a voice and body that go with the face. CP2 interviews the instant character. Say, "I know you have been writing monologues and creating characters. But since we still don't know what our play is going to be, we may need a lot of new characters. This is a fast way to get NEW characters."

- *Deeper Dialogue, or "I want, I need, I feel":* Improvised scene-work for more emotional performance. Participants play a scene and take turns speaking as Character A and Character B. The lines must start with "I want," then "I need," then "I feel" in that order. Say, "Good dialogue makes it easier to act. So, we are going to practice with three powerful phrases that connect actors to their emotions: I want, I need, and I feel." Ask for two volunteers on stage. Give the instructions. Ask them to practice one time, trading the line sequence back and forth, just "I want, I need, I feel." When they are ready, seat them in chairs and say, "You are co-workers on a fifteen-minute lunch break. Remember that each of your lines will start with one of our powerful phrases."

Presenting Familiar Material as Performance: Participants have been generating material and building up expectations about the play for several weeks. CP2 should view a presentation of some familiar material to make it clear that all material from the group is being used, that participants are writing and creating, and that all levels of contribution are being accepted. Spend a minimum of 30 minutes considering material the group has already created. CP2 must have a response to each piece of work, including two levels of feedback. Say, "Thank you! What I noticed about that piece was ... ." And "it makes me want to ask the question: ... ." Say, "I know you have been getting ready for the weekend, and I want to share in some of the work you've been doing. What can we look at together now?" Look at three to five pieces of material.

- Working in advance with CP1, draft a list of one to three scenes that the group created and enjoyed. This may be read from scripts or memorized or re-improvised, but it should be performed from "onstage" with CP2 sitting in the "audience."
- Working in advance with CP1, choose two to three monologues from previous exercises. Consider a monologue from homework or from a session that was NOT expanded upon in earlier work.
- Ask the group to share any special skills that they hope to incorporate into the play. Participants may have a desire to sing, to dance, to play an instrument, or to do a particular trick. They may wish to make costumes or sets, and will say so here. Where possible, prompt the participant to SHOW the special skill rather than talk about it.

Closing

- Prepare participants for the intensive schedule, including meal preparation and transportation.
- *Thunderous Applause:* Each participant crosses the stage alone while the audience engages in thunderous applause. Say, "There is one last secret to

a great play, and it is the applause at the end. In fact, for the rest of this weekend, if you want something to be over, simply say 'The End,' and our group will give you a round of applause. No matter what. Practice it now – 'The End'". The group will applaud. Then say, "To bring us to a close right now, each one of you will cross the stage. Before you start, say 'The End,' and the group will applaud for you all the way across."

Movement Scorecard (MS) for CoATT

General Instructions

The team should decide who will score the MS based on the research design. Options include the individual delivering the intervention and/or an outside rater trained in CoATT. If the MS is being filled out by the individual delivering the intervention, the MS should be filled out directly after session for fidelity purposes. If a task scores less than a 2, it should be denoted and described in the protocol notes section at the end of the MS.

The following scale should be used to rate the degree to which the warm-up was completed by circling the number.

0 ······ Concept/exercise was not delivered by the practitioner

1 ······ Concept/exercise was partially delivered by the practitioner

2 ······ Concept/exercise was fully delivered by the practitioner

Movement	Intensive A
Duration	Three continuous sessions (Intensive A, B, C)
Facilitated by	CP2
Session Length	Flexible depending on participants needs
Overview	Master performance skills to match material created in generation
Participant Task	Learn theater skills, assessment, and training in service of the production
Participant Commitment	"We commit to working as part of an acting ensemble in collaboration with our co-active team"
Practitioner Task	Inspire confidence and develop resilience through teaching theater skills
Homework	Rest and self care

Date: _____

WARM-UP

Introduce CP 2 as a theater maker	0	1	2
Share participant commitment	0	1	2

CORE

Facilitate 1 to 3 of theater assessment exercises	0	1	2
Facilitate 3 to 5 spontaneous material exercises			
Watch 1 to 3 pieces of prepared material			

CLOSING

Facilitate self care discussion	0	1	2

Homework given: ☐ Yes ☐ No

Notes for manualization exercises not fully executed:

CoATT Practitioner: _____

MS completed by: _____

Role to project: _____

Figure 4.7 Movement Four, "Intensive A" scorecard for CoATT.

Intensive B

Who: CP2

Overview: Participants develop sustained theatrical expression in service of scripting a first draft.

Participant Commitment: "We commit to working as part of an acting ensemble in collaboration with our co-active team"

Participant Task: Participants develop sustained theatrical expression in service of scripting a first draft.

Practitioner Task: Generate unified material that connects characters and situations in service of the play.

Exercises

Warm-up: Bring the group together to prepare for sustained creativity and mutual support. Depending on the population, you may have developed a ritual warm-up. If so, begin with that. You may repeat any warm-up activity from previous sessions, including the previous Intensive session 6a. Deliver three to five focus and concentration games that include, but are not limited to:

- Sound and Movement
- Warm-up Walks
- Postcard from the Future
- Zip Zap Zop
- Mirroring
- 18 Entrance Lines
- What happened next?
- Stage Pictures

Core: CP2 leads the generation, exploration, and refinement of material that will become the first draft of the script. Since writing and notes may be generated, this session may require notebooks and pencils, that pre-printed scenes be read and marked up, or it may require ways to capture improvisation. Participants should be encouraged to improvise and work through material on their feet, though, rather than "write together" wherever possible. Highly functioning groups may choose to work in independent groups to develop and present new ideas. Divide the time between these:

- Lead at least two, but no more than four improvisational rehearsals of previously established scenes. Working with CP1, CP2 should have a list of scenes that the group already knows and can develop further.

  - Using improvisation, investigate how these scenes may extend to include other characters. Identify key moments of action in scenes and create "what happens next" additions. Consider creating scenes based on "What came before?"

- Explore assigning participants to new roles that CP1 and CP2 agree are most relevant to the recovery journey of that participant.
- Consider how the same character or characters appear in the different scenes.

- Develop a sequence for existing scenes.

  - If they were placed on a timeline, determine which scenes are first, and which scenes should follow. Participants can improvise monologues or short scenes to connect existing material.
  - Use an existing scene to launch a "hero's journey" for one character, in which that performer becomes the center of a narrative in which they leave home in search of something and return home changed by the journey. CP2 may want to lead this exercise for more than one character. Participants may play the same characters they have been exploring, or someone entirely new.
  - Take a monologue that has a story in it and make it into scenes with action instead of description.

- Create at least two (but as many as are needed) new scenes to support the evolving narrative. CP1 and CP2 may have developed a narrative idea based on earlier works from the group. These ideas should be explored with new scenes for familiar characters, or for new characters entering a completely new scene.

  - Improvise an opening scene that starts a journey.
  - Improvise a closing scene that reunites all characters.

- At least two ensemble sequences:

  - Create a Talking Tableau that sets the scene.
  - Create a movement piece involving all participants.
  - Create an environment with sound effects created by the participants.
  - Create a song or score with instruments provided by and played by participants; instruments may be improvised.
  - Improvise a large meal or banquet for all characters.
  - Create a ritual that defines the world of the play.

Closing: Do both exercises.

- *Conversation on the Script:* Say, "In our next meeting, we will gather to read our first draft. I want to thank you for everything that you've contributed. I also want to remind you ahead of time – that the script will be a draft. There will be things you love and things you don't like. Our job will be to accept this draft as a starting point and commit to making it the script we want to share with the audience."

Movement Scorecard (MS) for CoATT

General Instructions

The team should decide who will score the MS based on the research design. Options include the individual delivering the intervention and/or an outside rater trained in CoATT. If the MS is being filled out by the individual delivering the intervention, the MS should be filled out directly after session for fidelity purposes. If a task scores less than a 2, it should be denoted and described in the protocol notes section at the end of the MS.

The following scale should be used to rate the degree to which the warm-up was completed by circling the number.

0 ······· Concept/exercise was not delivered by the practitioner

1 ······· Concept/exercise was partially delivered by the practitioner

2 ······· Concept/exercise was fully delivered by the practitioner

Movement	Intensive B
Duration	Three continuous sessions (Intensive A, B, C)
Facilitated by	CP2
Session Length	Flexible depending on participants needs
Overview	Participants develop sustained theatrical expression in service of scripting a first draft
Participant Task	Share material and work in support of one another's dramatic reality
Participant Commitment	"We commit to working as part of an acting ensemble in collaboration with our co-active team"
Practitioner Task	Generate unified material that connects characters and situations in service of the play
Homework	Practice self-care

Date: _____

WARM-UP

Share participant commitment	0	1	2
Facilitate 3-5 focus and concentration theater games	0	1	2
	0	1	2

CORE

Facilitate at least 2 but no more than 4 improvisational rehearsals of previously established pieces	0	1	2
Facilitate at least 2 but as many new scenes as needed to support the evolving narrative			
Facilitate at least 2 ensemble pieces			

CLOSING

Facilitate conversation in the script reveal	0	1	2
Facilitate Future Audiences exercise			

Homework given: ☐ Yes   ☐ No

Notes for manualization exercises not fully executed:

CoATT Practitioner: _____

MS completed by: _____

Role to project: _____

Figure 4.8 Movement Four, "Intensive B" scorecard for CoATT.

- *Future Audiences:* Place a chair for each participant in audience rows. Ask each participant to take a seat. Participants will embody future audiences. Say, "As we start to imagine doing the play, we might start to imagine how an audience will respond. So, in a moment, I will ask you to show me what three different audiences are like." Give three prompts. Say, "Show me an audience that hates the play." Then say, "Show me an audience that loves the play." Then say, "Now take a moment to answer this question: From your own point of view, how would you like an audience to feel if we do the play just as you are imagining it? Show me that audience."

Intensive C

Who: CP1 & CP2

Overview: Present and accept the first draft of the script in service of a fully realized production.

Participant Commitment: "We commit to nurturing the script and growing it into the story we want to tell."

Participant Task: Begin to flesh out the script and roles as related to individual and group recovery processes.

Practitioner Task: Tolerate the fear, anger, and disappointment of the cast upon script reading.

Exercises

Warm-up

1 Share and embody the participant commitment
2 CORE:
3 Seat the group in a circle, pass out the script, and assign roles.

   a Read the play
   b Collect responses and suggestions for rewrites
   c Begin connecting the play to themes and recovery

Closing

1 Commitment to fix the play (you may only change your own lines).
2 Repeat the Participant Commitment in embodied form.

Movement Five: Rehearsals

The first meeting during Movement Five requires the cast to solidify the script before rehearsing begins. Thus you will notice below a delineation between first and second meetings.

Movement Five, First Meeting

Duration: 1 session

Who: CP1

Participant Task: Arrive at an agreed-upon script that is the vehicle for a theme of recovery that the group is exploring through performance. This

Movement Scorecard (MS) for CoATT

General Instructions

The team should decide who will score the MS based on the research design. Options include the individual delivering the intervention and/or an outside rater trained in CoATT. If the MS is being filled out by the individual delivering the intervention, the MS should be filled out directly after session for fidelity purposes. If a task scores less than a 2, it should be denoted and described in the protocol notes section at the end of the MS.

The following scale should be used to rate the degree to which the warm-up was completed by circling the number.

0 ······ Concept/exercise was not delivered by
the practitioner

1 ······ Concept/exercise was partially delivered by
the practitioner

2 ······ Concept/exercise was fully delivered by
the practitioner

Movement	Intensive C
Duration	Three continuous sessions (Intensive A, B, C)
Facilitated by	CP2
Session Length	Flexible depending on participants needs
Overview	Present and accept first draft of the script in service of a fully realized production
Participant Task	Tolerate the fear, anger, and disappointment of the cast upon script reading. Begin to flesh out the script and roles as related to individual and group recovery process.
Participant Commitment	"We commit to nurturing the script and growing it into what we feel our story is to tell"
Practitioner Task	Tolerate the fear, anger, and disappointment of the cast upon script reading.
Homework	Begin making edits to the script

Date: _____

WARM-UP

Share participant commitment	0	1	2
Assign roles and share script	0	1	2
	0	1	2

CORE

Read the play as a group	0	1	2
Facilitate discussion in relating the script to recovery and overarching theme selected			

CLOSING

Explain guidelines for making edits to the script	0	1	2
	0	1	2

Homework given: ☐ Yes ☐ No

Notes for manualization exercises not fully executed:

CoATT Practitioner: _____

MS completed by: _____

Role to project: _____

Figure 4.9 Movement Four, "Intensive C" scorecard for CoATT.

should be in service of sharing with an audience, and in service of bolstering individual and group recovery.

Commitment: We will use our strengths to bring our story to life and will examine how our fictionalized script and roles relate to our recovery.

Exercises

Warm-up

1   Support group members in leading warm-up of choice.
2   Share Participant Commitment

Core: Participants come to week seven with their suggested edits for their characters' words. We work through the script to arrive at an agreed script and title and read through the play again, and, if time permits, begin working on initial blocking.

Closing: Support cast in developing closing exercises to be repeated each week.

Therapist Task: Support participants in script changes and challenge directions that are not recovery-focused.

Homework: Write about how the role is like you and not like you. What change do you hope to see in the character you are playing?

Movement Five, Subsequent Meetings

Duration: 4–8 weeks, depending on the needs of the group (complete one scorecard for each meeting)

Who: CP1

Overview: Participants practice for the appropriate number of weeks needed to make a public presentation of the play in service of strengthening their recovery and sharing with an audience.

Participant Commitment: "We will use our strengths to bring our story to life and examine how our fictional script and roles relate to our recovery process."

Participant Task: Arrive at an agreed-upon script. Master the performance of individual scenes and roles. Rehearse and refine the production. Support each other in active recovery and overall group health.

CP Task: Support recovery by demonstrating the process of rehearsing a play and show how it parallels independent recovery.

Exercises

Warm-up: In the rehearsal movement, the group elects a participant to lead the warm-up each session. This can be any warm-up the group has used before and may stay the same or change from week to week.

Core

1   Learn to present the play as it will be seen by an audience. This includes the qualities of the performance, the text of the script, and the presentation of

Movement Scorecard (MS) for CoATT

General Instructions

The team should decide who will score the MS based on the research design. Options include the individual delivering the intervention and/or an outside rater trained in CoATT. If the MS is being filled out by the individual delivering the intervention, the MS should be filled out directly after session for fidelity purposes. If a task scores less than a 2, it should be denoted and described in the protocol notes section at the end of the MS.

The following scale should be used to rate the degree to which the warm-up was completed by circling the number.

0 ······ Concept/exercise was not delivered by the practitioner

1 ······ Concept/exercise was partially delivered by the practitioner

2 ······ Concept/exercise was fully delivered by the practitioner

Movement	Rehearsal*
Duration	4–8 weeks (complete one scorecard for each meeting)
Facilitated by	CP1
Session Length	2 hours
Overview	Participants practice for any number of weeks needed in order to make a public presentation of the play in service of strengthening their recovery and sharing with an audience.
Participant Task	Arrive at an agreed upon script. Master the performance of individual scenes and roles. Rehearse and refine the production. Support each other in active recovery and own group health.
Participant Commitment	"We will use our strengths to bring our story to life and examine how our fictional script and roles relates to our recovery process."
Practitioner Task	Support recovery through demonstrating the process of rehearsing a play and parallels to independent recovery.
Homework	Ongoing self care and preparation for production

Date: _____

WARM-UP

Support group member in leading warm up of choice	0	1	2
Share participant commitment	0	1	2
	0	1	2

CORE

Practice the presentation of the play	0	1	2
*One week of rehearsal, design co-active element	NA	Y	N

CLOSING

Support cast in developing closing exercise to be repeated each week	0	1	2
	0	1	2

Homework given: ☐ Yes   ☐ No

Notes for manualization exercises not fully executed:

CoATT Practitioner: _____

MS completed by: _____

Role to project: _____

Figure 4.10 Movement Five scorecard for CoATT.

the material. Presentations may include any theatrical elements such as lighting, sets, or costumes as long as the presentation is public.

2   One week during rehearsal, the cast will design the co-active element. Please see the previous chapter for details.

Closing: The group develops a closing exercise that they will repeat each week (Figure 4.10).

Movement Six: Performance

Duration: One run of 1–3 performances

Who: CP1 and CP2

Overview: A public performance that includes audience members in a co-active element in service of answering the CoATT question.

Participant Commitment: "I commit to standing in my recovery and sharing a worthwhile perspective with my community."

Participant Task: Present a fully realized production as related to the theme that answers the question: "What is a theme of recovery that we want to explore in service of strengthening our recovery, and that we want to share with an audience?" Include the audience in a co-active element.

CP Task: Ensure technical aspects of the production are secured. Provide support for the cast and facilitate participants supporting one another. Introduce the performance.

Exercises

Warm-up: Engage in the ritual warm-up previously agreed upon by the group.

Core

- Support the participants in performing the play.
- The audience and the participants complete the co-active audience element.
- Engage in real-time processing of feelings, lessons learned, and accomplishments throughout the process and relate these to recovery and chosen theme.

Closing

1 De-role.
2 Engage with the audience through post-show refreshments.
3 Gather after refreshments to check in.

Homework: Journal about what you are taking away from the process of a fully realized production that you co-actively created (Figure 4.11).

Movement Scorecard (MS) for CoATT

General Instructions

The team should decide who will score the MS based on the research design. Options include the individual delivering the intervention and/or an outside rater trained in CoATT. If the MS is being filled out by the individual delivering the intervention, the MS should be filled out directly after session for fidelity purposes. If a task scores less than a 2, it should be denoted and described in the protocol notes section at the end of the MS.

The following scale should be used to rate the degree to which the warm-up was completed by circling the number.

0 ······· Concept/exercise was not delivered by the practitioner

1 ······· Concept/exercise was partially delivered by the practitioner

2 ······· Concept/exercise was fully delivered by the practitioner

Movement	Performance
Duration	One run of 1–3 performances
Facilitated by	CP1 & CP2
Session Length	Variable
Overview	A public performance which includes audience tmembers in a coactive element in service of answering the CoATT question.
Participant Task	Present a fully realized production as related to the theme that answers the question: what is a theme of recovery that we want to explore in service of strengthening our recovery and sharing with an audience?" Include the audience in a co-active element.
Participant Commitment	"I commit to standing in my recovery and sharing a worthwhile perspective with my community."
Practitioner Task	Ensure technical aspects of the production. Provide support for the cast and facilitate participants supporting one another. Introduce the performance.
Homework	Journal about what you are taking away from the process of a fully realized production that you co-actively created.

Date: _____

WARM-UP

Share participant commitment	0	1	2
Oversee ritual warm up takes place	0	1	2
	0	1	2

CORE

Support participants in performing play	0	1	2
Support participants and audience in CoActive element	NA	Y	N

CLOSING

Lead clients in de-role exercise	0	1	2

Homework given: ☐ Yes ☐ No

Notes for manualization exercises not fully executed:

CoATT Practitioner: _____

MS completed by: _____

Role to project: _____

Figure 4.11 Movement Six scorecard for CoATT.

Movement Seven: Launch

Duration: As many sessions as needed to process (complete one scorecard for each meeting)

Who: CP1

Overview: Meaning-making, closure, and memorializing the process.

Participant Commitment: "I will contribute to my community as fully as possible in my active recovery."

Participant Task: Reflect and integrate processes and use the experience to set concrete goals. Using wisdom from the play, demonstrate support for how concrete goals will be addressed.

CP Task: Support goal-setting and meaning-making connections. Contact relevant treatment team members to support transition.

Exercises

Warm-up: The group does not warm up, but joins in a circle to discuss the end of the experience.

Core

1 Look at the artifacts from the Co-active element and reflect. Discuss: "What do you think the audience took away? What did you take away?"
2 Claim lessons from the play and the rehearsal process that will help support recovery in the future.
3 Discuss one concrete goal you will set based on what you learned from the play.
4 Plan a cast party to celebrate.

Closing

1 Say, "I am going to give you your final script in this process. When it is your turn say, "I did a play called _____ and played a character named_____ and the most important thing I learned is_____."
2 The participants take a final bow and clap.

A Word About CoATT Productions

In the following chapters, we discuss two different types of recovery, and two CoATT plays. In each chapter, we provide a brief overview of the diagnosis at hand, general recovery as understood by the mainstream mental health community, including typical treatment approaches and special considerations we have encountered in putting on a production with the identified population. These sections are in no way meant to be comprehensive but, rather, should be considered a framework to guide your considerations of our work with the

Movement Scorecard (MS) for CoATT

General Instructions

The team should decide who will score the MS based on the research design. Options include the individual delivering the intervention and/or an outside rater trained in CoATT. If the MS is being filled out by the individual delivering the intervention, the MS should be filled out directly after session for fidelity purposes. If a task scores less than a 2, it should be denoted and described in the protocol notes section at the end of the MS.

The following scale should be used to rate the degree to which the warm-up was completed by circling the number.

0 ⋯⋯ Concept/exercise was not delivered by
         the practitioner

1 ⋯⋯ Concept/exercise was partially delivered by
         the practitioner

2 ⋯⋯ Concept/exercise was fully delivered by
         the practitioner

Movement	Launch
Duration	As many as needed to process (complete one scorecard for each meeting)
Facilitated by	CP1
Session Length	2 hours
Overview	
Participant Task	Meaning-making, closure, and memorializing the process.
Participant Commitment	"I will contribute to my community as fully as possible, while working my recovery as the basis for my new identity."
Practitioner Task	Support goal setting and meaning making connections. Contact relevant treatment team members to support transition.
Homework	Complete any required assessments

Date: _____

WARM-UP

Share participant commitment	0	1	2
	0	1	2
	0	1	2

CORE

Review coactive artifact	0	1	2
Support participants in claiming lessons from the process			
Support cast party planning			
Connect lessons from the play to setting at least one concrete goal			

CLOSING

Deliver closing exercise	0	1	2

Homework given: ☐ Yes   ☐ No

Notes for manualization exercises not fully executed:

CoATT Practitioner: _____

MS completed by: _____

Role to project: _____

Figure 4.12 Movement Seven scorecard for CoATT.

chosen recovery population. We then present a close reading of the script, which highlights how the structure of the play relates directly to manualized exercises.

To appreciate the therapeutic journey and the process of recovery for a group, each character and scene must be analyzed through the lenses of the director, therapist, and dramaturg. These familiar roles from the theatre-making process use the same skillset employed by CP1 and CP2, as well as participants who are coactive in the creation of the play. As a director, one reads the scene for content and for elements of themes that are relevant to each performer, as well as to those that further the message of the play. As a dramaturg, one reads with an eye for the purpose and structure of the play. The inner dramaturgs ask if the work of the group is distributed in line with the CoATT principle stating that all material is shared and that the actors speak the words of other contributors. Additionally, the dramaturgical lens explores the forward motion of each character in terms of action and development. Finally, the therapeutic lens considers the way the script shows how the group is moving toward recovery. First, read the play with your director hat on, then come to the play and notation chapter with your dramaturgical notebook ready. Finally, read the whole chapter with your therapist lens present.

We close each chapter with details about the CoATT interactive element that was designed and facilitated by the specific recovery group. This includes additional movement notations to be aware of, and a presentation of relevant results or studies that have been conducted. Finally, we conclude by integrating the CoATT experience with the larger treatment continuum.

Note

1   This movement can be viewed online at: https://www.youtube.com/watch?v=8VhGgiowPuI. (NYU Theater and Health Lab , 2021).

Reference List

Brandt, A. M. (1978). Racism and research: the case of the Tuskegee Syphilis Study. *Hastings center report*, 21–29.

Cassiello-Robbins, C., Dietch, J. R., Mochrie, K. D., Elbogen, E., & Rosenthal, M. Z. (2022). When does modifying the protocol go too far? Considerations for implementing evidence-based treatment in practice. *The American Psychologist*, 77(7): 853–867. 10.1037/amp0000993

Drisko, J. W., & Grady, M. D. (2019). *Evidence-based practice in clinical social work*. Springer. 10.1007/978-3-030-15224-6

Fulford, K. W., & Howse, K. (1993). Ethics of research with psychiatric patients: principles, problems and the primary responsibilities of researchers. *Journal of Medical Ethics*, 19(2): 85–91.

Leavy, P. (Ed.). (2017). *Handbook of arts-based research*. Guilford.

NYU Steinhardt Theatre and Health Lab. (2021, January 6.) *Role theory and method: Co-Active Therapeutic Theater (CoATT)*. [Video]. Youtube. https://www.youtube.com/watch?v=8VhGgiowPuI

Truijens, F., Zühlke-van Hulzen, L., & Vanheule, S. (2019). To manualize, or not to manualize: Is that still the question? A systematic review of empirical evidence for manual superiority in psychological treatment. *Journal of Clinical Psychology*, 75(3): 329 10.1002/jclp.22712

Chapter 5

Eating Disorder Recovery

Introduction

The first population that CoATT worked with, and in many ways was inspired by, were clients in eating disorder recovery. This population is notoriously challenging, and the need for novel treatment approaches to sustain recovery is essential. For clients with eating disorders, the first year after higher levels of treatment is a critical period in which to support recovery, as it also marks the highest likelihood of relapse. CoATT productions provide clients with eating disorders a necessary space through aesthetic distance to continue to work on recovery, while also building new relationships to replace the primary relationship with the eating disorder.

Below, we discuss the production of *Twin Falls*, which took place in Saint Louis, Missouri in 2015 at the Gaslight Theatre. We picked this script because it highlighted several aspects that will support readers in seeing the principles of the CoATT model come to life.

Eating Disorders

Eating disorders, as defined by the DSM V include: Anorexia Nervosa (AN), Bulimia Nervosa (BN), Binge Eating Disorder (BED), and Otherwise Specified Feeding and Eating Disorder (OSFED) (American Psychiatric Association, 2013). AN "is characterized by distorted body image and excessive dieting that leads to severe weight loss with a pathological fear of becoming fat" (p. 171). BN is "characterized by frequent episodes of binge eating followed by inappropriate behaviors such as self-induced vomiting to avoid weight gain" (p. 172). BED "is defined as recurring episodes of eating significantly more food in a short period of time than most people would eat under similar circumstances, with episodes marked by feelings of lack of control" (p. 174). "OSFED is an overarching diagnosis for eating disorders that contain characteristics of AN, BN, and BED but do not fully meet the diagnostic criteria. OSFED is associated with marked distress and occurs at least once a week over three months" (p. 175).

Eating disorders are complex biopsychosocial disorders and often are comorbidly diagnosed alongside anxiety disorders, depressive disorders, and

DOI: 10.4324/9781003161608-6

post-traumatic stress disorder. Eating disorders are often seen as chronic, are further complicated by high relapse rates, and are challenging to treat, given that, unlike other addictions, one cannot be abstinent from food (Pinto et al., 2006). As Jones et al. (2005) confirmed, "Unfortunately, our ability to predict the course of eating disorders, to treat them efficiently and effectively prevent relapse remains limited" (p. 237).

Wilson et al. (2007) noted that the need for non-medical interventions for eating disorders was essential to treatment success, for maintaining recovery, and particularly essential in identifying "mechanisms (mediators) of thera-peutic change" (p. 212).

Eating Disorder Recovery

One of the most challenging issues facing the eating disorder treatment com-munity is the struggle for professionals to operationalize "a clear, consistent, and measurable definition of recovery from eating disorders. ... We can't assess something which is not clearly defined" (Noordenbos, 2011b, p. 447). Qualitative and quantitative research on recovery has, at a minimum, concluded that recovery must be defined as more than just a reduction of eating disorder symptoms and must also include a wide spectrum of a person's quality of life and capacity to engage in the world (Noordenbos, 2011a; 2011b; Wood, 2016). Noordenbos (2011b) conducted a comprehensive qualitative study delineating 11 areas that must be addressed to constitute recovery. These included eating and drinking, physical activity and exercise, attitude toward food, body eva-luation, physical recovery, psychological recovery, emotional regulation, relax-ation, social relations, sexuality, and treatment of outstanding comorbidities.

Treatment As Usual

Eating disorder treatment in the United States typically offers five levels of care: inpatient, residential, partial hospitalization, intensive outpatient, and out-patient. Each level of care is scaffolded to support clients in moving from more oversight of eating disorder behaviors to more autonomy in treatment (Wood et al., 2022). At the inpatient level, the primary focus is on the stabilization of the body and attending to the physical harm that has taken place because of the eating disorder. Residential treatment begins to pair physical recovery with psychological recovery, but clients are still highly monitored around their meal plans and eating disorder behaviors. At the partial hospitalization level, clients are still provided significant care, but they are beginning to work toward more autonomy and freedom around food and body choices. Upon entering inten-sive outpatient, clients are working on entering back into the world and are taking on more responsibility for the oversight of their recovery.

Despite working through the levels of care, clients with eating disorders have high chronicity, and therefore, require a long-term multidisciplinary approach. In their comprehensive literature review, Wonderlich et al. (2012) noted that a recovery-based model where a range of interventions are included may be most effective for this challenging population. Among those recommendations are a focus on empowerment and self-directedness, along with "the promotion of culturally appropriate independence in relationship to family, the development of strong support systems, the stabilization of symptoms and improvement of social skills, and the enhancement of strengths while minimizing deficits" (p. 6).

Considerations with CoATT and EDs

As the model was initially conceived and inspired by this population, few, if any, modifications to the model itself are needed. There are other considerations beyond the manualization that are unique to eating disorders that may be important to discuss with the team and make decisions around, with the most obvious being the schedule of eating, snacks, and proper hydration. The theatre, in general, does not necessarily make its schedules and lifestyle conducive to recovery, so addressing this directly is important. For all the productions we have done with clients in eating disorder recovery, we offer a peer-supported meal prior to the start of rehearsal. Participants are forthcoming about what snacks they need to be eating and take responsibility for asking for a break and time to eat them. The Intensive also prioritizes an eating and hydration schedule. A positive relationship with movement and embodiment is core to eating disorder recovery, making drama therapy, in general, quite powerful. A heightened awareness of the use of the body, costumes, and other physical elements of theatre is needed when considering a CoATT production with clients in eating disorder recovery.

Production: Twin Falls

Twin Falls is a CoATT script that contains clear examples of the intention and the process of applying the CoATT model post-treatment. The group that created this production was notable as a cohort for several reasons. First, the group was among one of the most "purely homogenous" groups that we worked with using the model. Second, because all participants were in treatment together, they had a shared language, understanding, and experience with "drama therapy" and "eating disorder recovery." Finally, the group contained members who had previous experience in the CoATT model. As a result, the manualized processes were implemented directly, and produced clear and compelling outputs apparent in the script and the moment of production.

In terms of group makeup, this cohort presented with an eating disorder as the primary diagnosis for treatment. As with most eating disorder patients, there were complicating dual diagnoses and a wealth of historical circumstances that compounded the complexities of group dynamics and individual treatment. As individuals, though, they came together with a shared focus on their eating disorders and with the clear understanding that this treatment was intended to support recovery from eating disorders. This dynamic supports the intention of the CoATT model, which is bridging the gap for people who are in treatment for trauma or addiction and who will eventually reintegrate back into their community.

There were seven participants in Twin Falls: six women and one man, ranging in age from 23 to 33 years old. Each participant is described in this section based on the information from the demographic questionnaire and from the published dissertation study by Wood (2016). The names used here are pseudonyms.

Participants

Callie was a 24-year-old who identified as a White, heterosexual woman. She was single and had never been married. She earned some college credits before entering treatment. At the time of the interview process after the performance, she was gainfully employed part-time as well as attending college again. She identified her family as being from an upper-middle-class socioeconomic background. She was in recovery from BN and BED and had also been diagnosed with clinical anxiety and depression. At the start of the project, she had been discharged from treatment for approximately three months. Before the start of the project, though, she had been in higher levels of eating disorder care on three separate occasions. Callie had lost her mother to cancer when she was a young teenager, and the unresolved feelings from this relationship were often present in the current manifestation of her eating disorder. Coming into the project, she had no acting experience.

Sidney was a 32-year-old who identified as a White, heterosexual single woman. Before the project, she had been in treatment twice – once for two months and then again for nine and a half months. At the start of the project, she was two and a half months out of treatment and was struggling. She was diagnosed with BN, AN, and orthorexia, as well as with bipolar disorder and post-traumatic stress disorder. At the time of the interview, she was in out-patient treatment and employed part-time.

Raj was a 33-year-old who identified as an Asian man. He was divorced and had earned his bachelor's degree. He was raised upper middle class and diagnosed with BED, anxiety, depression, and post-traumatic stress disorder. At the time of the project, he was self-employed and working on a men's clothing line for larger-sized men, as inspired by his work in recovery. He was in treatment once prior to the play and was also a member of the previous CoATT production. At the start of the study, he was 11 months into his recovery.

Piper was a 31-year-old self-identified White woman. She was divorced and described her sexual orientation as pansexual. She grew up lower-middle-class and, at the time of the project, was receiving Social Security disability assistance. Coming into the project, she had earned some college credit. She was diagnosed with OSFED, dissociative identity disorder, post-traumatic stress disorder, and anxiety. She was four months out of treatment at the start of the project and had been in treatment 14 times. Post-project, she started college and was in outpatient treatment. Prior to the project, she had theatre experience, but no therapeutic theatre experience.

Victoria was a 25-year-old who self-identified as a White, single, hetero-sexual woman. At the time of the project, she was one month into recovery after intensive treatment. She had completed her bachelor's degree and was raised in an upper-middle-class family. She was diagnosed with BN, depression, and anxiety. She had a musical background, but through the course of her eating disorder, had lost passion and connection to her musical abilities. She was enrolled in a master's program and in outpatient treatment.

Ellie was a 31-year-old single, White, heterosexual female. She had a master's degree in occupational therapy and, post-project, she was self-employed and worked as a nanny for kids with special needs. She grew up lower-middle-class and was diagnosed with AN, major depressive disorder, generalized anxiety disorder, obsessive-compulsive disorder, post-traumatic stress disorder, and dissociative identity disorder. Prior to the project, she had four admissions to residential eating disorder treatment.

Charmaine declined to turn in her optional demographic form but shared in groups that she dated women and had been in eating disorder treatment multiple times. She was employed full-time at a coffee shop and babysat on the weekends.

The two returning members of the project reinforced the power and importance of the model in the minds of the other performers. Notably, neither participant had experienced relapse for more than a year, so both could attest to the benefits (and the intensity) of the performance experience. Each of them had the chance to explore new roles as mentors and role models while also exploring character roles that gave depth to their journey in recovery. The presence of the returning actors influenced the theme and the structure of the script and elevated the sense of commitment and value for others.

Excerpt and Commentary

The strength of the *Twin Falls* script lies in the cohesive and powerful way that the group responded to the CoATT Question. Their answer gave us the central metaphor, as well as the tools to unpack it through narrative. The answer begins grounded in the eating disorder diagnosis that everyone in the group shared. They also shared the idea that if the eating disorder makes you feel perfect, like a god, we can portray that statement through our main characters. Pushing past the characterization of eating disorder and toward the principles of recovery delivered the theme: When you let go of the god-like feeling of the eating disorder, you are left with being "only human," and all the enormous feelings, pains, and joys that come along with humanity. The clarity of both answers came from the deep and shared experiences of both the disorder and the treatment. This commonality of language and theory allowed the group to explore multiple paths of recovery, as well as the multiple protective functions of the disorder. Ultimately, the process of making a play together, and presenting it to the public launched group members into their long-term recovery with a community of like-minded supporters found in both the treatment community and the community at large. Perhaps the most generous offer made in the entire process was to the audience: Share our humanness to share our recovery.

TWIN FALLS
_____

ACT I

The Facade

AT RISE: Lights up on a Roman fresco. In the middle are TWIN GODDESSES, SYLVIA and STEVIA – fraternal twins, standing on two theatre blocks, both draped in beautiful togas. In their hair are laurel wreaths. At their feet reclines a handsome man, PLASTINO, also in a toga, holding a goblet of wine and a platter of delicious organic fruit. Around his head a crown of grapevines and clusters of grapes. On either side are two HANDMAIDS, each in togas, both holding hand mirrors, which the TWIN GODDESSES stare into. On each of the edges of the stage tableaux are two other goddesses, SPORTIVA and ATHLETA: One has a tape measure wrapped around her waist and across her chest, the other is flexed holding golden barbells, one in each hand. **(1)**

PLASTINO

Long ago

ATHLETA

In the past

SPORTIVA

Long long ago

PLASTINO

Long ago in the past

HANDMAIDEN 1

In the past

HANDMAIDEN 2

In the past

1 Act 1 of *Twin Falls* presents a tableau and prologue to the play that firmly establishes the intent of the production. The classical fresco tableau is an embodiment that emerged in the Intensive weekend. The group quickly arrived at the message of the play, which was an answer to the key question, "What do you want people to know about Recovery?" The answer for this group was: "When you have an eating disorder, you think that you are perfect. It's a god-like state. Once you give up your eating disorder, it's like being a regular human with vulnerability and pain." Everyone in the group could relate to that concept, so they created a tableau of "the gods" as they might exist in a perfect state. Together, we crafted a poem about that perfect state, and the opening of the play was established.

SPORTIVA

In the past

ALL (but TWINS)

The gods were perfect

TWINS (together)

No matter what, things are perfect

PLASTINO

And, there is wine. So much wine.

TWINS (together)

And that's just perfect.

ATHLETA

And food ... delicious organic, gluten-free, dairy-free, low-carb whole food

SPORTIVA

To keep us "healthy"

HANDMAIDEN 1 and 2

And always beautiful

TWINS (together)

And it's just perfect

PLASTINO

Long ago, in the past, there were twin goddesses.

TWINS (together)

Fraternal twins!

PLASTINO

They were royalty among the gods. Everyone took care of them. Not because they were beautiful, although they were ...

TWINS (together)

Thank you!

PLASTINO

Not because they were perfect **(2)**

HANDMAIDEN 1

Though you certainly are.

2 There are several elements of the tableau that advance the recovery of group members. Most notably, the tableau asks for confidence in the presentation of each individual body. Further, the chorus speaks of the bodies as beautiful while looking in mirrors and wearing togas. This strong and positive body awareness is a sign of recovery and stands in direct opposition to body dysmorphia and to the compulsive control of one's image that usually mark eating disorders. Regarding the male participant in the tableau, he had arranged himself reclined on the ground with a knee raised, and his torso angled to the audience as the god Plastino. This was a chance to assert his sexuality and desirability in a rehearsal setting. He noted that one of his goals in recovery was to have a stable and healthy romantic relationship with a woman. He noted that he did, in fact, have sex appeal and could, perhaps, bring that quality into his life beyond treatment. This authentic investment in portraying the character existed in the dichotomy of naming the character Plastino, which was meant to invoke the shallow and hard surface of cheap perfectionism.

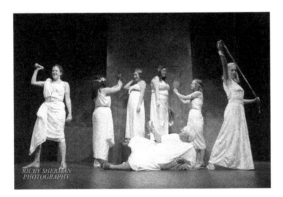

Figure 5.1 The cast of *Twin Falls* creates the opening tableau of the heavens. Photograph by Ricky Sherman Photography.

                    HANDMAIDEN 2
Indeed.

                    TWINS (together)
Thank you!

                    PLASTINO
And not because they were perfectly in control of everything that happened. And everything that anyone
thought about them.

                    ATHLETA
Though you certainly are.

                    TWINS (together)
Thank you!

                    PLASTINO
But simply because they were daughters of the God Ed **(3)**

                    ATHLETA
Ed, the all powerful!

                    SPORTIVA
Ed, the soothing!

                    STEVIA
Ed, the perfect father!

                    SYLVIA
Who loved the perfect mother!

                    HANDMAIDEN 1
Ed, the all knowing!

                    HANDMAIDEN 2
Ed, the god of secrets!

                    PLASTINO
But - Ed the God did have a secret. Though his daughters
didn't know it.
        (PAUSE)
Long ago, one dark night his craving overtook him

                    ATHLETA
He went down to earth, he couldn't stop himself

3   The tableau also serves as a starting point for the action of the play. It establishes the perfect, ideal state from which our heroes will be cast out. It creates the sense of home and harmony that an "ideal recovery" might promise, while also dramatizing the false sense of perfection that the eating disorder protects. In the text, the group makes the most overt statement about eating disorders to be found in the story but does so by establishing a central metaphor: the father figure, who is called Ed (short for "eating disorder," and a common shorthand in recovery circles), and who is made all-powerful. The god Ed sets the rules and insists on perfection. It is important to note that the god Ed is also responsible for the fall of our heroes; he has strayed from perfection and permitted humanity to pollute the very existence of his children.

SPORTIVA
and he saw a beautiful girl, a human.

HANDMAIDEN 1
not a goddess at all, but a human!

HANDMAIDEN 2
Vulnerable, naive, soft, and human. Really human.

TWINS (together)
What happened?! What did he do!?

PLASTINO
The woman was in pain, and he showed up and whisked her away, and brought her here, and made her a goddess queen.

TWINS (together)
Our mother?!?!?!

ATHLETA
You're only humans!

SPORTIVA
They are only human?

HANDMAIDEN 1
Nothing but humans!

HANDMAIDEN 2
You're not goddesses! **(4)**

PLASTINO
With a flaw like this we must cast you

ALL
OUT!

(Goes to dark. We hear the sound of the girls make a long fall)

GIRLS
Ahhhhhhhhhhhhhhhhhhhhhhhhhhhhhhhhhhhhhhhhhhhhhhhhh.

(Cast clears stage during this time) **(4)**

(END OF ACT I)

4   Dramaturgically, the tableau efficiently jumpstarts the play. We present the main theme using a metaphor that comes from the shared language of recovery found in this cohort, dramatize the double bind of perfection/isolation that the eating disorder creates, introduce our main characters, and begin the action by expelling our heroes from their home due to a tragic flaw. From a therapy perspective, we also establish the safety of the group, who are presenting themselves powerfully and all at once, which allows them to show their expertise in the subject matter and display the artistry that is helping them develop a life in recovery. In line with the CoATT model, the use of metaphor prevents the "after-school special" dynamic of "a play about eating disorders presented by survivors." American audiences will remember these television specials, which gave cursory attention to serious issues with maudlin and abbreviated consideration of very serious topics.

ACT II

THE FALL (5)

AT RISE: A loud thud. Lights up on the girls
                            in a pile on the ground.

                            STEVIA

Ow!

                            SYLVIA

Ow! OWWWW!!!

                            STEVIA

Ohh Ohh Ouuuuuu

                            SYLVIA

OHHHH OHHHH

                            STEVIA

Wahhhhhh!!!!! Dad!!!!!!!

                            SYLVIA

What is this?

                            STEVIA

I don't know - it ... hurts!

                            SYLVIA

Hurts? This ... I've heard of this ... this is pain.

                            STEVIA

What's that? It sounds terrible!

                            SYLVIA

Well, that's what happens when you get kicked out of your
home. It hurts. You and I have never felt that before.

                            STEVIA

Ohh feelings. FEELINGS!!!!

5 The transition into Act 2 is contained in a stage direction that offers a glimpse into the ways that traditional drama therapy supports therapeutic progress. Our heroes, Stevia and Sylvia, are asked to pantomime a long fall from the skies to the earth, complete with a long theatrical "ahhhhhhhhh," and mimed with the physical comedy of pratfalls. This small moment afforded real growth for both performers. To create this effect, the actor has to use the body fully and extremely, while making a long and loud supported sound. For many trauma survivors, sustained physical investment, taking up large amounts of space, drawing attention to oneself, allowing laughter at one's body, and giving into the physicality of a scene partner can be challenging. Our rehearsal for the moment was nearly 30 minutes long, leaving both actors and CP2 exhausted and panting on the floor. Indeed, at that point in rehearsal, the participants have become actors. So, physical and vocal warm-ups are as important as an emotional warm-up to the material.

Act 2 of *Twin Falls* demonstrates the way writing prompts from the homework come to be woven into the script. These are preferably spoken by a cast member other than the author. The ensemble was eager to share the full range of emotions encountered in treatment and was determined to support the recovery of each individual in the group. Rehearsal became an action psychotherapy group. This ensemble was also quite committed to poking fun at and making critiques of the eating disorder treatment community, as well as their treatment center. Both CP1 and 2, well-versed in inpatient treatment settings, recognize this healthy assertion of self and boundaries that differentiate the person from the patient role. The play script accommodates this through humor as a way of respectful rebellion.

                              TWINS (together)
Journal! **(6)**

                    (They pull out their journals from their togas
                    and speed write. After a moment ...)

                              SYLVIA
Thank god we kept these. Never go anywhere without it.

                              STEVIA
I know.

                              SYLVIA
What did you write?

                    (STEVIA opens her journal and reads.)

                              STEVIA
That fall was so scary. I don't feel like I can go on. But I
have to. I have to risk everything and trust that it won't
go to shit. I'm terrified. I'm literally on a cliff and its
crumbling around me and I need to jump to the other cliff –
but I'm not sure it's any safer and it might crumble after
I land on it - or I might not even make the jump at all. I
want to go back to dad.

                              SYLVIA
Well ... you're not literally on a cliff ...
                              STEVIA
Shut up. What did you write?

                              SYLVIA
It's so different here. Everything is dark around me. I
feel the darkness closing in. What was once clear is now
hazy, muddled and distorted. This place is nothing like
home. I don't think we can stop here. We might sink. It all
came crashing down around me. We have to keep moving.

                              STEVIA
That's so good. It's better than mine.

                              SYLVIA
No its not! Yours is better.

                              STEVIA
No yours!

6 "Feelings!" is the horrified prompt for "Journal!," and gives the script another recovery joke. In treatment, patients are constantly asked to share feelings, face feelings, or work with their feelings. Feelings can be perceived as the enemy, as such a source of pain that a person could die from them, and indeed, much of eating disorder behavior is an attempt to manage or numb feelings away. After intensive treatment, patients begin to understand that feelings are a natural part of the human experience. They gain practice dealing with their feelings in healthy and expressive ways and may come to see the fear and pressure around their feelings as both manageable and comic. In rehearsal, the twins wrote the lines and got to play out their new relationship to feelings. Once our heroes land on Earth, they begin to experience pain, at first physically, and then emotionally. To cope, they shout at each other, "Journal!" and open notebooks to record their new thoughts and feelings. Journaling is a technique used in the treatment center and is also used in the CoATT model to great success. Patients in treatment, though, often criticize tools for being too simple or failing to contain the unique pain or struggle they feel. Dr. Wood notes that some people use the journal as a shield or distraction from engagement, particularly in Expressive Therapy groups. She forbids journals in the group. There's a hint of collusion in this repeated joke. The participants in the group get to make fun of the technique and feel more connected to Dr. Wood in the process. More importantly, they give a voice to a feeling many people in early recovery experience when confronted with slogans, steps, or techniques that promote change. At the same time, the characters they play do benefit from journaling, and the participants continue to use journaling as they participate in the process. The joke promotes a healthy ambiguity, which is necessary to a life in recovery.

                    SYLVIA
No!

                    STEVIA
No!

                    SYLVIA
No. YOURS! **(7)**

                    STEVIA
What are we going to do!!!

        (She drops to her knees, fists hit the ground)

                    SYLVIA
I don't know. But let's keep moving. I can't just sit here
with your feelings

                    STEVIA
Or yours!

                    SYLVIA
Fine. Or mine! Let's go.

        (They start walking)

                    SYLVIA
Left right left right left right

                    STEVIA
Fine! Ugh!

                    SYLVIA
Left right left right

                    STEVIA
I get it. Ok.

        (SYLVIA rolls her eyes. They come to a street
        corner.)

                    SYLVIA
Stop.

                    STEVIA
What is it?

7 Another dynamic from treatment that emerges from journal writing comes when the twin heroes immediately share and compare journal entries. In group treatment, particularly for eating disorders, patients may develop a competitive relationship with others in the cohort. Early on, this may manifest as a sort of contest for who had the "worst eating disorder" or "did the most shocking or horrifying thing" as part of addiction or active eating disorder. Competition may be just as strong when presenting "the best recovery" or "strongest program." As with all group treatment, some element of competition for the love and attention of the therapist is at play. In *Twin Falls*, the heroines reinforce the emotional experience of the other by downplaying their own journal entries to point out the low self-esteem that many people in recovery face when moving away from the disorder or addiction.

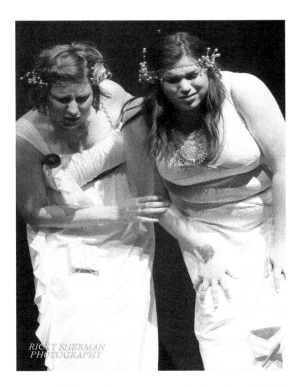

Figure 5.2 Two goddesses come to Earth in *Twin Falls*. Photograph by Ricky Sherman Photography.

SYLVIA

It appears to be some kind of ground made of blackness and
filth. This small cliff seems to separate us from it. But I
see there is another cliff on the other side, there by
that blinking light.

STEVIA

The yellow one?

SYLVIA

Well..yes..but now its red. Come on.

> (We hear horns. Loud. The TWINS scream. And run to
> the other edge of the stage. They are frazzled and
> overwhelmed from the traffic. They are now in front
> of a pushcart of food. There is water, snacks,
> fruit, etc. It says, "Ms. Waits's Yums Yums." MS.
> WAITS is on the backside of the cart stocking the
> shelves and or sweeping.)

STEVIA

I'm feeling something.

SYLVIA

What?

STEVIA

I don't know. It's just ... something big. In my stomach.

TWINS (together)

Journal!

> (They take out their journals and they pause and
> they are stuck.)

SYLVIA

(getting angry)
It's not working! It's not enough.

STEVIA

It always works. We've always journaled since we were
kids and it's always worked.

SYLVIA

Yeah. Well. It's not working now. Whose idea was journaling anyways?
(Grabs the box of hostess cakes.) **(8)**

STEVIA

What are you doing?

8   When the positive coping tool of journaling fails to provide relief, one of the twins reaches for a snack to soothe the feelings. The Hostess Cupcakes are found on a pushcart of food that offers an array of choices. Here, we see the basic eating disorder behavior demonstrated, but not commented upon. In fact, the action has immediate consequences that propel the story forward. The ensemble approached the play with a clear sense that the disorder was something deeper than bad eating habits and talked openly in group and rehearsal about the misconceptions around an eating disorder. By this point in treatment, all the members of the ensemble were able to illustrate behavioral examples of what an eating-disordered patient might *do,* while aiming to reveal something deeper about how a person in recovery might *feel.*

SYLVIA

I don't even know ... but it feels like eating this will
make me feel better.

STEVIA

Well gimme one too.
    (They open the boxes.)

MS. WAITS

Excuse me, but you haven't paid for that yet! **(9)**

SYLVIA

What do you mean?

MS. WAITS **(10)**
    (with sarcasm)
Money. Ever heard of it?

SYLVIA

No.

MS. WAITS
    (more sarcasm, with some rudeness)
Well I don't know where you're from, but here on planet
Earth, when people need food. They pay for it.

TWINS (together)
EARTH! We're on earth!!!
    (They start off excited, they have figured it out,
    yelling, jumping, celebrating, and then it turns
    to panic and anxiety, "Holy shit, we are on
    Earth—what are we going to do?!")

STEVIA

This is terrible!!

MS. WAITS

Yeah, no shit. Welcome to my world. That's life in the big
city for ya.

SYLVIA

I don't like it here. It's nothing but pain, loud noises
and missing home.

9   In this case, the reach for Hostess Cupcakes gets the heroes into trouble. They've broken the law by shoplifting from Ms. Waits' Yum Yum Cart. This small crime moves us away from the world of eating disorder treatment and pushes us forward in the story. We introduce a set of characters that show how hard the world can be for those who don't have "the protection" of their eating disorder. Ms. Waits introduces the twins to real-life consequences and stressors. She also speaks directly to the loneliness and isolation that everyone faces, the kind of overwhelming sensitivity that informs the inner life of many people with eating disorders. By the end of the act, the twins have also met Ursline, a street-living runaway making bad choices just to stay alive.

10 Character names carry special meaning and importance for writers and performers, sometimes sending an important message to the audience. In *Twin Falls*, the ensemble was scrupulous about naming, taking ownership over every detail of the writing. There were good laughs around the Yum Yum Cart, and it was also tied to the personal history of one participant. As mentioned, the god Plastino was named to indicate shallow and shiny perfection. Ms. Waits took her poignant name as a summation of the inner monologues she speaks in Act 2, both of which were taken from journal writing and character writing in earlier CoATT movements. The character takes two different journal entries and explains to the twins (and to the audience) some of the darkest and hardest feelings in recovery. In one speech, she describes the way a patient must confront the reality of their unmet dreams and frustrated wishes. In another, she details the frustration of trying to build healthy relationships in the new world of recovery. Both themes focus not on the eating disorder, but on the recovery journey, and both dynamics are most often treated with the same wisdom: it takes time. A lot of recovery is waiting for the healing to happen, and Ms. Waits is trapped in those painful moments. So, she waits.

MS. WAITS

I know what you mean. I'm not from here originally. Where I came from it use to be either sunshine and rainbows or complete and utter shit. For the longest time I thought that people were either good or bad and ideas were either right or wrong. There was no room for negotiation. A favorite motto of mine was "go big or go home." So I came here, to the big city. It was such a shock when I landed here, you know? I honestly figured the city would be either heaven or hell. Floating among fluffy white clouds or dodging pits of lava. But no. It's not black or white here. Its grey. The dullest shade of fucking grey. It's funny, people spend their entire lives being saints to avoid not ending up in hell. But to be frank with you. I think the in between is worse. **(11)**

SYLVIA

Well that sounds terrible.

STEVIA

Why would anyone want to ever be here?

MS. WAITS

Ah, well, you can't change the past. This is where I ended up.

SYLVIA

Can you change the future?

MS. WAITS

Maybe.

STEVIA

Good. Please change ours.

MS. WAITS

Are you two sisters or something?

STEVIA

We are! Twins. **(11)**

MS. WAITS

You don't look like twins

TWINS (together)

We're fraternal.

11 Both women playing the twins were ready to take on leading roles, and each seemed poised to learn something from playing the full journey of a hero story. The idea that they would play sisters (or twins!) was a practical way to incorporate two leads. While one woman was working through themes of maturing into womanhood without a healthy mother figure, the other was working through gender and sexuality in hopes of building a safe romantic life. For the first character, we wanted to suggest a beautiful and idealized "leading lady," and so suggested the name Sylvia with all the languid beautiful associations it carries. Our second lead tried on many matching names including Salvia and Serena. Ultimately, she arrived at the choice of Stevia, which carried for her both genders in the name Steve. CP2 noted that Stevia is an alternative sweetener, highlighting the subconscious ways that themes around eating disorders continue to present themselves well into recovery.

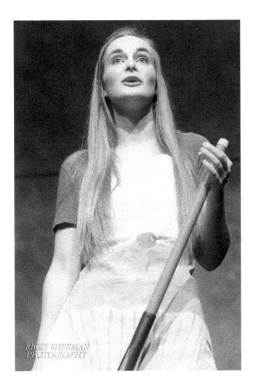

Figure 5.3 Ms. Waits struggles to tolerate everyday emotions in a soliloquy. Photograph by Ricky Sherman Photography.

(A street urchin teen, URSLINE, enters in, she
licks her lips. She's hungry and desperate.)

MS. WAITS

Oh that's a surprise. Life is full of surprises, that's
for sure. Guess that's one thing about life in the big
city. Here ... Gimme those boxes back. Take these.

(MS. WAITS hands them each a bottle of water, then
and apple and each a cupcake.)

I don't know if I can change the future. But maybe this
will make your day a little easier.

URSLINE

Oh, hey. I'm with them, too. Can I have some?

MS. WAITS

Oh, well..sure.

(She turns around to get another bottle of water. The
street urchin grabs arms fulls of food and yells.)

URSLINE

Run! ! ! !

(The girls are confused, panicked and afraid so
they run. MS. WAITS is alone.)

MS. WAITS

Stop! Not again. Damn it. I'm exhausted. I took a risk by
reaching out and this is what happens. I'm risked out. I
want to be brave and connect to people, but instead I find
myself tired and worn down. Maybe I'm better off alone. I
should stop chasing after people and connection because
more often than not, once I catch them, I find myself com-
pulsively caretaking them anyway. I won't talk about my
feelings or me. I fall into a black hole and I don't exist.
Maybe I should stop and I'm tired of chasing them anyways.
I wish I could find my home. **(12)**

(BLACKOUT)

(END OF ACT II)

12 Structurally, Act 2 of *Twin Falls* treats the theme of the play by placing the characters deeply in the problem they will face: living as an imperfect human. The dramaturg might see this as creating a strong journey for our heroes. They should find themselves as far away from the solution as the story will allow. *Twin Falls* shows us physical suffering, isolation, loneliness, bad behavior, and even despair. There is real misery in the scene despite the comic energy, and the ensemble worked hard to present the reality of the play. In staging, we gave Ms. Waits an old broom and cleared a lonely space for her to share her shattered dream. The actress used the image from Les Misérables of Cosette, left alone imagining a castle in the sky, to help her channel the simple but emotional truth of the scene. This performer had expressed worry about bringing emotion to a public performance and was adamant that she wanted to take a minor role. Ms. Waits had a manageable amount of text and included material that was wry and bitter, funny, and ultimately vulnerable. Working with the support of scene partners helped to launch her performance, and space alone on the stage helped her to share her vulnerability. Her therapeutic growth focused on facing a self-imposed limitation, taking a healthy risk, and being part of the ensemble. Her performance contribution was important, but her role as a member of the group and ensemble was equally powerful.

Naturally, a play about recovery will retrace the steps that the group has taken together on their collective recovery journey. Each act of *Twin Falls* has a title that tracks to the recovery journey, and each references a dynamic in treatment at the center. This stems from the fact that this cohort had a strong set of shared experiences in recovery, as well as a shared vocabulary. For most groups, this is difficult to achieve unless their recovery is built under similar circumstances. *Twin Falls* presents "The Façade" and "The Fall" to establish a metaphor for eating disorder and recovery, followed by "Finding yourself, finding others" as the first beat in the story that speaks to the difficulties of recovery. This section extends the discussion toward the topic of treatment, and why recovery is challenging, as opposed to why an eating disorder happens and how the disease manifests. Ms. Waits' speech that leads into this section became a point in supervision for CP1 and CP2; intense work with eating disorder patients can be demanding, and draining, and may induce feelings of hopelessness. The feeling of being used up and cast aside or wanting to give up on a relationship altogether is familiar to therapists. Projective identification with this material in supervision led to real-time intervention in the rehearsal room. CP1 raised the dynamic by asking, "What is different about healthy relationships in recovery?" She followed this with the question, "How are we practicing balanced and healthy relationships in this work?" Real-time reflection on this reinforced the respect and boundaries established as ensemble members, underlined the nature of healthy support for others that includes detachment, and highlighted the sense of hope, optimism, and future that must accompany the creation of a public performance. Ms. Waits' final speech aligns the script, and therefore the cast, with the experience of the audience, or at least those in the audience who have suffered at the hands of a loved one with an eating disorder. This transformation of feelings from the specific struggle of early recovery to the universal feelings of frustration and despair in the face of disappointing relationships is a primary aim of the CoATT model. Participants are reintegrating into the world at large through shared experiences and understandings.

ACT III

<u>FINDING YOURSELF, FINDING OTHERS</u>
(13)

AT RISE: Sound of sirens Lights up on the
                    three.

URSLINE

That was awesome!!! How was the party? **(14)**

STEVIA

Excuse me?

URSLINE

Aren't you dressed up for a costume party? How are drunk
are you?

SYLVIA

We're not drunk.

STEVIA

We're twins.

URSLINE

You don't look like twins ...

TWINS (together)

Fraternal!

URSLINE

You're going to a fraternity party? Can I come?

STEVIA

Ok!

SYLVIA

We don't know where we are going.

URSLINE

Me neither. But I know I'm not going back there.

SYLVIA

Wait—did you just steal those?

URSLINE

Yeah. So what. I'm homeless and broke.

13   "Finding yourself, finding others" can be read as a microcosm of group therapy. Three participants find themselves thrown into intimate circumstances. They try out their identities with each other and get candid feedback. Our heroes claim their goddess status, but Ursline easily deflates their sense of specialness and power. Ursline is challenged on her criminal behavior and offers what might be her standard defenses, but the twins push back and hold her to a higher standard. More importantly, as the three struggle toward intimacy, they cause each other pain. Ursline's pain becomes the basis of identification and connection.

14   Ursline the street kid took her name from the word "urchin," and feminized it. The name was suggested by CP2 and prompted a telling therapeutic discussion. The ensemble member had joined the CoATT group due to her interest in performance and her desire to be a professional singer. She also held herself apart from the group, declining the supported eating sessions and arriving just on time for rehearsal with no socializing. She sat apart in the rehearsals and treated the drama therapy work as straightforward theatre games. When asked what roles she was best suited to play, she answered, "the Disney princesses." Yet when given the character name Ursline, she commented that it was "like Ursula, the Sea Witch." CP2 offered to change the character name, but the actor declined, stating "it's perfect for me." The actress, who most readily describes herself as a princess (the way others see her), sees her inner self as an evil and overweight witch. Characters in a play can be a projective objective (as distinct from 'role') that gives enough aesthetic distance to work with both senses of self. Ursline causes trouble for everyone, demonstrating a common theme in recovery groups. When someone with an eating disorder must commit dangerous, hurtful, and shocking actions in order to survive with their disease, families and communities begin to see that person as problematic. They are often the black sheep or negative star, wreaking havoc like tornadoes touching down in the lives of the people around them. Ursline has done just that.

SYLVIA

Yeah, well, we're homeless and we don't steal.

URSLINE

Well it's different. I was thrown out of my home.

STEVIA

Well, we were too. And we don't steal. Come on Sylvia, let's get out of here.

URSLINE

Fine with me. Do whatever you want. I'm gonna be a big ol' star in Hollywood one day and you'll see my name in lights.

STEVIA

So what?

SYLVIA

We are goddesses!

STEVIA

Real goddesses.

URSLINE

Yeah, then snap your fingers and make all my dreams come true.

SYLVIA

Why should we?

(Before she can answer STEVIA jumps in and snaps her fingers.)

SYLVIA
(under her breath)
Or ... were anyway ...

URSLINE

Nothing happenin'. Look like mortals to me.

SYLVIA

Shut up!

(SYLVIA pushes URSLINE, she falls.)

URSLINE

Ouch!! Owwwww!!!!

(URSLINE starts to cry. SYLVIA and SALVIA pause.
They remember their fall. They step back. They
drop to their knees.)

STEVIA

That's pain, isn't it!

URSLINE

Leave me alone! Leave me alone!!! What kinds of goddesses
are you? Leave me alone.

SYLVIA

Its hurts, doesn't it? I'm so..sorry ... I'm sorry!

STEVIA

I'm sorry, too!

URSLINE

Just leave me alone!

STEVIA

No. You are a star.

URSLINE

No I'm not. But ... I will be. Just wait, you'll see!

STEVIA

Show us.

SYLVIA

We wanna see you.

(URSLINE sings her song, she's nervous at first,
but gains confidence as she goes and sings and acts
the shit out of the number. As people walk by they
give her money. The song is heartbreaking, beautiful, and hopeful; the twins are moved.) **(15)**

STEVIA

That was amazing!

SYLVIA

So beautiful.

15   When Ursline sings on the street corner, that identification deepens into appreciation. The intimate relationship with the twins, based on shared needs, allows her to show not just her dreams, but her special skills and talents as well. She is truly seen, supported, and encouraged by the twins. Her positive presentation of self is rewarded with money that helps solve an immediate problem, rewarded as well with connection that launches her onto a better path. The twins "want to see her" and "believe in" her. She's found a substitute behavior, singing, that makes her forget her pain and feel like herself again. She has renewed purpose.

This sequence is a self-contained scene that was primarily built to give the ensemble member playing Ursline a chance to sing, so the parallel with her treatment is obvious. The song choice, "Only Hope" (Moore, 2015) was not so obvious. The song had personal meaning for the actress and provided material to discuss regarding romantic attachments and trust.

Building it into a narrative flow that helps to develop our theme, and making certain to show change and growth in the twins as well, is critical for the progress of the group in the CoATT model. Real-time reflection with the actresses playing the twins helped to ground the song choice for the production. For the ensemble, the song pointed out how young the goddess characters felt and reminded them all that we were placing them in a world that closely resembled our real-time world because it was contemporary. Most members of the group did have struggles around romance and trust, and several had been young people on the street to varying degrees. For DT2, who had little to no familiarity or interest in the song, the group process around the song was a point of co-active collaboration. This choice made the play the work of the group and not the idea or sole creation of the therapist.

URSLINE

Thanks. When I sing, I forget for a moment all the hurt in my past and I just feel like the real me, ya know?

SYLVIA

I know what you mean ... but to be honest, I'm not even sure who the real me is anymore ...

STEVIA

Me either. Or what it means to be real ... So, what is all this stuff people put here?

URSLINE

Holy shit!!! That's a lot of money!

SYLVIA

You could pay back MS. Waits!

URSLINE

Why would I do that when I can finally make it out of here?

STEVIA

It's a different kind of feeling. Because when I pushed you, I remembered when people pushed me. And it made me feel terrible. But being with you now. I just feel ... connected ...

SYLVIA

You should try it.

URSLINE

I'm used to being pushed around and I'm pretty good at being alone and disconnected. Why would I want to do something so difficult? I'm still having trouble at seeing the possibility of a life without sacrificing parts of what I want and need. I'm scared, but I guess ... I'm willing to try. **(16)**

(They hold her hand or embrace. It is quiet for a moment.)

STEVIA

Good

(URSLINE turns to walk away)

SYLVIA

Hey, wait! What's your name?

16   The dialogue following the song demonstrates another way in which the CoATT model prioritizes co-creation. The characters need to have an emotional reaction to the song. It must move the progress of recovery forward in order to explore the theme, and it should move the action forward for all three characters. The easiest way to find that reaction might be to hear the song and improvise lines, but the script was due at the end of the weekend Intensive, and the actress had been unable, and somewhat unwilling, to choose a song. DT1 had the collected material of the Generation movement and was ready to create the scene. Using journal entries and creative writing assignments, CP2 was able to write the shape of the scene and the reactions in advance of selecting the song. This is an example of taking material from the entire group process and repositioning it to serve the function of the play. In other parts of the script, such as Ms. Waits's speeches, longer chunks of stand-alone ideas can be lifted and assigned to a character. Here, line-by-line or phrase-by-phrase cuts of material are pulled together into brief, but compelling dialogue. This approach to text is an idiosyncratic skill that CPs 1 and 2 must develop in order to work in the CoATT model. Both therapists must cultivate a finely tuned ear for the text of sessions and assignments. Therapists are always listening, of course, and often are listening for deeper meaning and emotion than is initially presented in the text. CoATT practitioners must also listen for compelling turns of phrase, metaphors, figures of speech, or flashes of ideas that can be culled into dialogue for the play. Capturing these in session notes is standard practice. Identifying texts by reading, re-reading, or in some cases, "coding" and cataloging, the creative assignments and journals not only enriches the therapeutic relationships in the group, but it also delivers the pieces that are used to make a play reflecting the totality of the groups wisdom and experience

URSLINE

Ursline. My name is Ursline.

SYLVIA

Good luck, Ursline.

STEVIA

I believe in you.

URSLINE

Me too.

(She exits) **(17)**

(END OF ACT III)

17 For Act 3 of *Twin Falls*, the dialogue captures several important emotional moments in a recovery journey. "I'm not even sure who the real me is anymore" and "when I pushed you, I remembered how it felt when people pushed me" came from different writers and assignments. Even within one sentence, "I'm used to being pushed around" and "I'm pretty good at being alone and disconnected" are combined from different sources to expand a feeling for the character. Other phrases such as, "Why would I do something so difficult?" capture the experience of early recovery, which for this group mirrored the dynamic at their treatment center. The suggestion to pay back Ms. Waits might be seen as making amends for bad behavior while trapped in the eating disorder. This scene leaves Ursline with a challenge for how she wants to move forward in her new life in recovery.

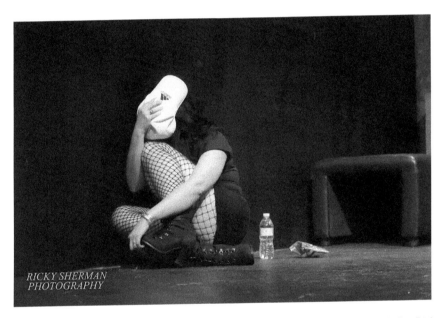

Figure 5.4 The street urchin Ursline, a character in *Twin Falls*. Photograph by Ricky Sherman.

<u>ACT IV</u>

<u>FORAGING AHEAD</u> **(18)**

TWINS (together)

Journal!!!

STEVIA

I'll go first! People can come together and be so creative and energetic and inspiring! It will take practice for it to become second nature but I'm going to challenge myself. Ok, you read yours!

SYLVIA

This is hard. It's different here. But I am still happy I'm pushing through, even though it's taking everything in me to not run away. But honestly, I wouldn't want to go back to my old life anyway. How could I go back to a perfect world knowing what I know now?

STEVIA

You wouldn't want to go back to our amazing life? Aren't you missing being perfect! It was so perfect!

SYLVIA

Was it? I can't even remember any more if that is true. The more I start to feel pain and connect to people and be in this world, it is like I am waking up for the first time. It feels so hard. But something about being here feels right. I feel ... alive.

BELLE

Hey, why are you guys dressed like that? Do you know Darrell? Looks like his style. You better watch out for that guy, he's not who he says he is.

SYLVIA

Is anyone?

BELLE

Hey, what are you guys doing out here? Are you working with Darrell?

STEVIA

Darrell???? No.

18 Note the pun in the title of this act. Although audiences didn't have access
to these titles, it was important for the cast to continue to be playful with
food imagery, demonstrating increased mental flexibility and humor.

In the structure of a five-act play, the characters and action are launched
in Act 1. Act 2 may feature a false solution to the problem they face, but it
sets them deeper into their quest. Act 3, the center of the play, offers a
crucial development that may allow the characters to resolve their conflict.
Act 4, most often, escalates the stakes of the story by moving all characters
forward toward resolution. In Act 5, the theme is advanced as the problem
gets resolved. This structure supports a focus on the journey of a hero
figure or figures. Crucially, every character we meet should have found
some resolution by this point. A change has occurred for all characters in
the story. Act IV suggests considering the progress of the play within the
same three lenses mentioned previously. At this stage, the dramaturg is
working to track the action of the play. The twin heroes have been
launched and the theme is established: It hurts to be human. Our heroes
made a friend who might have comforted them, but a complicated new
character sent them into deeper trouble. They made the important
discovery that shared pain is a crucial element of humanity. What might
happen that escalates the stakes? If the characters develop empathy for
others and healthy relationships, both actors and their characters feel more
invested in the successful resolution of their challenges.

The director is tracking the metaphor and material of the story:
Having an eating disorder was perfection because it transcended
human pain. The recovery journey is paralleled by the journey of our
goddesses through the human experience as they learn to encounter
and tolerate pain. The metaphor for human pain has come to life just
like the struggle to survive on the street, and we've seen four characters
struggling. They've discovered the secret that sharing pain is the key to
survival. What must resolve to restore their understanding of perfection? What change has happened to each character?

CPs 1 and 2 have been pulling material from multiple sources and have
been using journal entries and character writing that came from the second,
Generation movement. Real-time reflection has strengthened the recovery of
participants throughout and is reflected in the script. All participants have
appeared, but has each participant had the opportunity to create some
personal sense of change and growth? What needs to happen so that every
participant has the opportunity for transformation through the story?

For Act IV of *Twin Falls*, there were three ensemble members writing
character material that helped them to articulate deeper traumatic material.
As they were coping well with recovery, they were continuing to address
primary traumas. So, to raise the stakes in the story, their characters appear
and bring stories that illustrate some painful truths about being human.
These characters will also help to move the twin heroes forward on their
journey to balance pain with belonging.

SYLVIA

Never heard of him.

BELLE

You sure? Dressed like that (?) ... looks like his style. You better watch out for that guy, he's not what he says.

SYLVIA

Turns out, nothing is.

BELLE

You're telling me. Get this, awhile back, I answered an ad for a"street worker"; I was excited to finally use my degree in social work. So, the "boss" Darell told me to stand here, on this street corner. He said it was the best corner in town and had a pretty interesting dress code for the job. I should've known something was off. I wasn't sure what was great about it; it's a janky area if you ask me. But the people seemed nice; I thought I'd be able to help some of them. A lot of guys driving by that'd roll down their window and ask how I was doing, a few even asked how much? I'd just wave, "Doing great. Thanks for asking!" They always looked confused especially when I'd offer to tutor them or help with employment, stuff like that. Then some nun handed me a bag full of individually wrapped, colorful, weird-shaped balloons: "God bless and be safe"? Were they magical or dangerous of some-thing?? Were for me anyway, I'm allergic to latex. Darrel told me I had to remember to ask people their name. When I realized it was a phony ad in the paper, it was too late. Now I make sure that creep isn't tricking others. I watch this street like a hawk. I'm Belle, who are you? **(19)**

SYLVIA

I'm Sylvia

STEVIA

I'm Stevia

BELLE

Are you guys twins?

TWINS (together)

Yes!

19   Several group members had sexual trauma in their history, with some common elements in each of their stories. Abduction, betrayal, and trust figured into two of the participant stories. So, when the monologue for Belle emerged, it carried great resonance for the group. The character presents as almost impossibly naïve, an important element when thinking about the link between early sexual trauma and protective coping behaviors, such as an eating disorder. Belle has been tricked into a life on the streets and forced to "work for" a character we never meet called Darrell. Her assumption, based on the appearance of our heroes in their togas, is that they have met a similar fate, but Belle has found her power, and she is using it to care for others and to offer them protection and guidance. The speech is full of humor, including a story about misidentified free condoms that get treated like balloons. Belle isn't consciously telling jokes or lightening the mood, though. Instead, the character can be played as a woman with a mission. She's there to turn her experience and strength into hope and purpose. She shares her truth, and she can see the truth of the situation in which our heroes have found themselves. The strength of their bond lies in recognizing each other: Belle is the first to note that the twins are fraternal without being told (paying off a setup that runs through the earlier scenes), she's witnessed them help Ursline, and she can articulate the pain that they've just shared with each other in the journal.

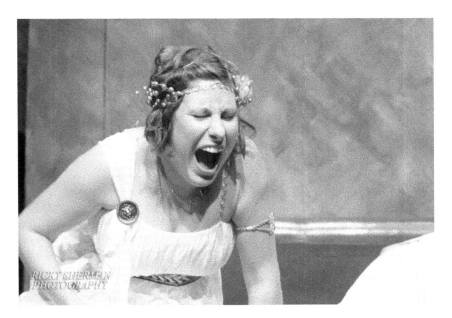

Figure 5.5 A goddess begins to understand human suffering in *Twin Falls*. Photograph by Ricky Sherman Photography.

BELLE

Fraternal, right? No judgment but ... your outfits come off as provocative, especially 'round here. Are you sure Darrell didn't send you ... you can tell me, it's ok.

SYLVIA

We don't know anything. We're just trying to get by. I guess we'd do anything to survive.

BELLE

You can make it without Darrell or the like. There are other ways.

STEVIA

We're not from here.

BELLE

I'll protect you. I know my way around nowadays. I had some bad things happen to me, but I'm smarter now and care a lot that it doesn't happen to others. I lost time in a haze of fear and avoidance getting out of some tough shit, then I just felt desperate and hated myself for it. I didn't want help from anyone, I was like an island of a person. I don't do that anymore. I found some really good people. I'm not afraid of living today or trusting the good in people. I can help.

SYLVIA

How do we know you're good? What if you are just working for this Darrell guy or someone else? Nothing on Earth seems trustworthy.

STEVIA

(quietly, pleadingly to SYLVIA)

But she wants to help us.

BELLE

Look, trusting someone is scary at first, sometimes ter-rifying, makes you want to crawl in a corner and hide. You don't have to come with me today, but I'd like to show you where I found help when I needed it. I saw what you did for that homeless girl. It takes guts to do what you believe is right, a lot of courage to listen to your heart and trust yourself. Life only gets harder when we push all the people away. There ARE good people around, like you, that want to help, nothing more. **(20)**

20 Audiences watching this scene in *Twin Falls* are getting a glimpse inside the recovery group. Belle employs the language of the treatment group. She gently encourages them with "You don't have to come with me today, but I'd like to show you where I found help." She assures them they are not alone, saying, "There are good people around like you who want to help," and before anything else, she tells them her own experience and says, "I had some bad things happen to me, but I'm smarter now and care a lot that it doesn't happen to others." This kind of deeply personal sharing and support is central to long-term recovery. Information, modeling, and instruction for healthy behavior, even identification, can happen in a formal setting. In recovery groups, however, there is no hierarchy or commercial interest. Community is built; intimacy is practiced in a safe space. The fact that all group members are equals and that there is mutual benefit, but no material to gain is, central to the power of twelve-step recovery. In *Twin Falls*, the dynamic unfolds on stage, explicitly.

As in life, the offer of help moves our heroes according to their own senses of their own struggle. In the moment that follows Belle's offer, Stevia responds to the hope and wants to go with Belle, but Sylvia can't trust people. It's the first moment in the play where the twins diverge. For this group, it was important to point out that recovery is individual and non-linear; not even twins will have the same kind of suffering or recovery. And so, there are no guarantees. For the actors sharing these roles, this role was a powerful intervention. The actor playing Stevia would be quick to point out that, in her real life, she had trouble trusting others. The actor playing Sylvia, on the other hand, would say that she struggled to make her own way without pleasing others, particularly those within her family. Each participant chose to take the path in the play that would be the opposite of their natural tendencies. Stevia convinces her sister to follow Belle to the place where they might find help in a moment that is powerful for those who deal with eating disorder and recovery. When asked how this moment mirrors recovery, the group recognizes the moment they decided to go into treatment. This moment of admitting that help is needed, and that others may be able to help, is central to the story of recovery. Belle helps both sisters in this moment as she shares her experience of recovery. Belle identifies feelings of fear and isolation, but she also identifies with the difficulty of trust and the hard work of letting other people into your suffering.

STEVIA

Come on, she's right ... we have nothing; nowhere else to go. I'm tired.

SYLVIA

Ok, lead the way.

> (Lights crossfade to the other side of the stage. TROY is standing there. He runs an animal shelter and is getting ready for dinner. He starts by bringing on a table and a few chairs. He goes back and gets a dog. He brings the dog out and starts to brush him. The moment the dog sees BELLE he barks and runs to her.)

(END OF ACT IV)

ACT V

FEELING AND FINDING YOURSELF (21)

BELLE

Hey Troy. I found two more strays.

TROY

No problem, There's always room for more.

STEVIA

We're not strays, we're twins.

SYLVIA

I can't believe you brought us to an animal shelter. We may not be goddesses but at least were human.

TROY

You don't look like twins.

BELLE and TWINS

Fraternal.

TROY

Oh, got it. Well I found a "stray" too. This is Ms. Waits.

MS. WAITS

I was really down on my luck and at my wits end and then I unexpectedly found money and a note saying, "I feel terrible for stealing from you, I know you were just trying to help and I took advantage of it. Please don't give up on the world, there are good people out there."

21   Act 5 is called "Feeling and Finding Yourself," which is an apt summation
of life in recovery as it continues beyond the treatment center. It is also no
coincidence that the two remaining group members were returning
veterans of a previous CoATT production. They came to the process in
a later phase of their recovery, intent on giving back to others who are
recovering from an eating disorder. They strongly believed in the benefits
of the model and saw participation as a way to maintain and strengthen
their own continuing recovery. So, the material they generated centered
around the rewards of living in recovery and maintaining health.
Integration of recovery principles and integration into society are the
key themes of Act 5. Here, they offer the warmth and the care for self and
others that are lost through eating disorder. The title of the act promises
the action of healthy adults. Where are these behaviors learned? Ideally, of
course, these are instilled in people by a good enough mother in childhood,
within the healthy biological family of origin. For many patients with an
eating disorder, that safe and balanced childhood is missing or damaged.
One image that recurs in drama therapy with people who live with eating
disorders is "the missing mother." As in fairy tales and Shakespeare, heroic
ingenues are left without a mother through death, remarriage, or
unexplained but dire circumstances. The search for the missing mother is
synonymous with the search for home; the promise of the good-enough
mother is to love and be loved.

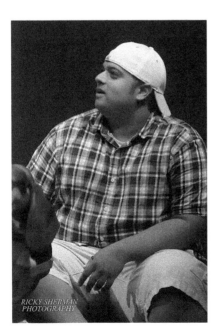

Figure 5.6 A man shares the story of his journey to community. Photograph by Ricky
Sherman Photography.

TROY

I was out on one of my daily dog walks and ran into Ms. Waits, who told me her story. I was so moved that I shared my story ... (22)

STEVIA

Sylvia!

SYLVIA

Shhh! Go on.

TROY

I was an only child growing up. A few years ago my mother passed away unexpectedly. But she always told me to follow my heart. At the time I had my best friend, Jupiter, a golden retriever mutt who was with me my entire life. However, he died around the same time my mother did. I was left alone, to live with my uncle and aunt. They weren't well off so I had to help in any way I could. I started working with my uncle at the factory nearby. Factory work was difficult. During my lunch breaks I would eat out on the railroad tracks. There was always a stray dog that would be outside meandering about looking for scraps. And every lunch break, I'd give half of my sandwich to a very eager and happy canine. I didn't know it at the time but within the next couple of weeks, my life would be forever changed. (23)

STEVIA

Sylvia!!! Its-

SYLVIA

Shhhh!!!!

TROY

You may call it sheer luck or God's touch or the universe picking me back up, but nothing would ever be the same. You see, on my 21st birthday, my uncle gave me a lottery ticket as my gift. A few weeks later, on my way to work, I passed the newsstand and saw that the winning ticket for 150 million dollars went unclaimed. Curiosity nagged me to take a look at my ticket and sure enough, I became the richest person in my town. I begged my uncle and aunt to take the money as gratitude for taking me in after my mom died. But they wouldn't have it. So, I followed my mom's advice, and I opened this animal rescue facility. With several volunteers, including my aunt and uncle, 1 set out to complete my life's work by helping as many dogs, and cats, that have been left without a home and unloved. But I learned there are just as many people who need the same thing. So, everyone is welcome to make a home here.

22   Ms. Waits has been integrated into this world of good-enough care. She reports that her money was returned, so we know that Ursline did the right thing at the urging of the twins. Further, we have the sense that this is where she would have sent the twins. When asked how this is like recovery, the group responded that "it takes all kinds of things, and some luck, to get into recovery." They know that they did not get to or through recovery on their own, and they wanted to demonstrate the many ways people might make their way to a recovery community. This is also notable through how Ms. Waits is in the final scene. When it was initially presented to her that she would be in the scene, she stated that it didn't feel realistic to her, that Ms. Waits doesn't get to have a good-enough ending. As the production continued, though, and as she built relationships with the cast, she began to internally feel she did deserve the support and the community. She came to rehearsal close to the opening of the show and shared that she felt Ms. Waits did in fact deserve to have a good-enough ending. In the model, cast members can re-write anything for themselves as long as it honors the integrity of the show and does not have to change other people's lines. An important recovery message is embedded here: You get the freedom and responsibility for your own actions in the world, not the actions of others.

23   Troy is discovered in a caregiving role, attending to a dog from his "home for lost things." He tells a story that begins with a missing mother and tells of how he learned to care for other living things. He's found a way to mother himself by integrating his mother's message: follow your heart. He's faced loss and suffering, yet has found purpose and meaning through sharing and helping. Notably, he shares food with the dog, Jupiter. He demonstrates that he has enough food and that he is making choices about food. He is using it as intended, to nurture and support. He also offers a nod to the "magic" of making it into recovery; he tells us it was luck, the love of his uncle, and his own will that got him to this place.

STEVIA

It was me!!!!
   (SYLVIA shakes her head.)

ALL

What? **(24)**

STEVIA
   (kneeling and takes his hand)
I know this sounds crazy. But I'm the reason you won the
lottery. I'm actually a goddess ... or was a goddess. I
watched you from above, grieve, work hard, have courage,
have fun playing with animals, being kind and be genuine
and I wondered: What must that be like? **(25)**

TROY

Come look at my place and I'll show you.

   (During this exchange, LITA, a beautiful and
   mysterious woman, has begun to set the table for
   dinner. She smiles when TROY takes STEVIA hand.)

LITA

So, that's two extra plates for dinner.

SYLVIA

I'm not sure I'm staying **(26)**

BELLE

Ok. I understand. You're free to go. But I want you know:
This is a safe place. And if you choose to, you can make it
good here.

   (TROY, STEVIA and BELLE exit.)

LITA

This is a good place to be. I came here with nothing. But I
found myself.

24 We also see how good acts that are put out into the world can return dividends. Sylvia and Stevia start to understand that it was their prompt (as humans) that helped get Ms. Waits money. Stevia realizes that it was her action (as a goddess) that got Troy his funding for the shelter. Stevia is able to take these signs of healthy living and good nature as portents of recovery. She and Troy become deeply connected, spending the rest of the play arm-in-arm. She's seen him, "grieve, have courage, work hard, have fun, be kind to animals ..." and she wants to know what that life could be like for her.

25 It wasn't easy to reach this resolution for Stevia. Even though it was taken from the writings and rehearsal with the cast, the staging of the moment where Stevia makes herself known to Troy was problematic for the actor portraying Stevia. DT2 wrote it in as a proposal on bended knee. Stevia couldn't play it that way; she was unwilling to kneel before a man because it was triggering and sent a disempowering message. She refused to link the two characters at all. So, it was rewritten to have no explanation for the lottery ticket. Then, the actor decided *she did* want it to be a moment of love and connection but did not want the kneeling. The cast supported this rewrite as well. Ultimately, the actors arrived at an action for the scene that allowed each to bow to the other on bended knee, showing a union of equals driven by mutual love and respect. Here, the CoATT model is seen in action, with the entire group deciding and directing the script and production.

26 Sylvia is less compelled by the stories of integration. The mysterious woman who appears to set the table for dinner holds a key to her chances for resolution and integration. The actor playing Sylvia had, herself, lost her mother and traced much of the insecurity and fear in her recovery to that childhood loss. The actress playing Lita, another of the returning veteran participants, was working through issues with parents as well. In particular, she was coping with an overbearing and controlling father who had a major impact on her safety in recovery, as well as with an absent mother who would not or could not help. The conversation between Sylvia and Lita was dense with possibilities for both actors.

SYLVIA

Well, I've got worse than nothing. I lost everything. I was thrown from my home. Chased through the city, scared and desperate. And now I might even lose my sister, at least that's what it feels like anyway.

LITA

I know something about loss. Many years ago, someone loved me so much; he came into my world to get me. I was sick, but I was also in love and ready to fight for this person. He helped me make a plan for my future; to return to my world he comforted me when things felt too much, he held me up when I could no longer stand. Until that connection became my burden and his hold on me became my crutch. I thought that as long as I did what he said was right, I ... would be fine, but I wasn't. I would be fine, but I wasn't. And his love wasn't enough to hold me up any longer. Love can't save you from your pain. It can help, but it can't be the only thing that you have. Eventually, you will need more. (She takes out her journal.) I wrote the story here so I would remember it. **(27)**

SYLVIA

And you had two beautiful daughters ... but you lied to them. And you left them. **(28)**

LITA

I did. But I didn't lie.

SYLVIA

You gave them a journal and left them alone and disappeared. They needed you.

LITA

No, I was sick. I did my best. I loved them and I never stopped.

SYLVIA

But love is not enough. You just said, love is not enough. But you fell and then they fell. They fell and they hurt, and they suffered. Fuck you.

LITA

I know. I'm sorry. It's ok that you are angry with me.

27   The "journal" prop and theme show the connection between lost mother and daughter quickly. The simple narrative explanation, however, is not presented as a solution to the big questions that are presented by our themes. DT1 determined in early sessions that "getting angry" would be a breakthrough for the actress playing Sylvia. The actress playing Lita stated that she wanted to feel stronger in her choice to be separate from her biological family at this stage of recovery. The scene wrote itself, deeply enriched through rehearsal with the actors.

28   The theme is restated with excruciating emphasis: To be human is to suffer. Additionally, the wisdom of this group in recovery, namely that sharing pain is the key to moving ahead in recovery, is also restated with personal stakes attached. The group would not settle for the easy resolution. Sylvia tests the wisdom with straightforward and truthful attacks. "You lied" is met with "I left but I didn't lie. "They needed you" is met with "I did my best." "Fuck you" is met with "I'm sorry. It's okay that you are angry .... " Here is the good-enough mother, offering a good-enough solution. Other people, fallible and with their baggage, are enough to help.

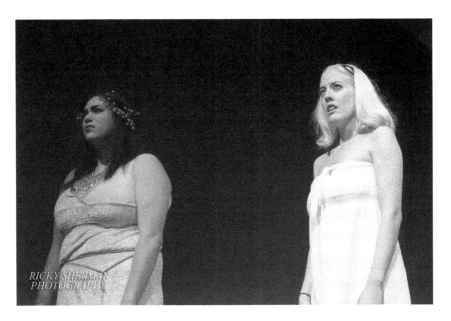

Figure 5.7 A goddess and her mother work through themes of rupture and repair. Photograph by Ricky Sherman Photography.

SYLVIA

But you weren't there. You weren't there when everyone fussed over me, and you weren't there when everyone turned on me. And I took care of Stevia. I did. That wasn't my job. I had to get us through it. You weren't there.

LITA

I'm here now. And you're here too. I'm sorry.

SYLVIA

How can you say that? Being here doesn't make up for it. You think I'm sorry is supposed to be enough? **(29)**

LITA

No, there's still a lot of work ahead us. I want you to know, I found people who cared so much that they stay here to be with me, they didn't push me back up, and they didn't try to save me. They listened to me and talked things out. They asked how they could help and were when I needed them. I may not have had someone to love me. But I had many who cared. And they aren't my crutch because I don't allow them to be. I knew I needed to get out. I could no longer rely on your father and that other world to save me. I needed to get out for me. And if you want, you can stay here and do the same. I hope you do.

(A beat)

SYLVIA

Can I help you set the table?

LITA

Are you going to break the dishes?

SYLVIA

I might. I'm really mad.

LITA

That's ok. There's more in the kitchen. **(30)**

(They set the table as the lights fade.)

(END OF PLAY)

29   Sylvia is a deeply realistic character. This can be seen as maturity; she's come as far as possible from the sheltered and childish goddess, removed from all suffering and reality. So, she's skeptical, saying, "You think I'm sorry is supposed to be enough?" Here, she's met with the deepest truth that the group can put forward: Hard work, done together, is what lies ahead. The only real promise that can be made, from one survivor to another, is the promise of help.

30   The tension of the moment is unresolved, but the answer to Lita's statement contains a clue that integration will win out. Sylvia can make the small step toward recovery when she asks, "Can I help you set the table?" Her move to become a person who helps is her real step toward recovery. She holds on to herself and her truth. She may break dishes because she is "really mad," and her good enough mother replies, "That's okay. There's more in the kitchen." She seems to suggest that recovery, and a group of people living in recovery, have enough resources to handle the damage of any one individual.

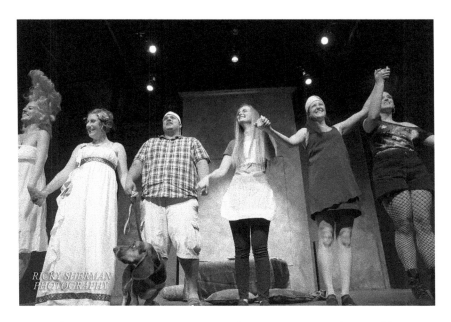

Figure 5.8 A proud cast takes their final bow. Photograph by Ricky Sherman Photography.

The CoATT Interactive Element

Participants in Twin Falls were excited to engage directly with the audience and took the opportunity to help audience members reflect seriously. After months of their own therapy, they were well primed to be enrolled as Expert, Facilitator, and Healthy One. Using the theme of journaling from the play, they asked audience members to journal: "What is the hardest part about embracing my own humanity?"

The cast was eager to read the responses right after the performance. They shuffled through all the index cards, sharing and reading aloud comments that felt particularly meaningful for them. The cards served as a tangible reminder of the impact their work had after the production. Furthermore, it facilitated a clear way to engage the audience in reflecting on the shared universal themes of the play and offered the audience a "script" to begin to engage with cast members in the lobby.

Results

The comprehensive results for this group can be found in *The Use of Therapeutic Theater in Supporting Clients in Eating Disorder Recovery After Intensive Treatment: A Qualitative Study* (Wood, 2016). This grounded theory study, drawing on a qualitative methodology but remaining grounded in the data (Strauss & Glazer, 2017), produced four observations concerning the benefits of using the CoATT Model with clients diagnosed with an eating disorder. Those observations included the CoATT Model's ability to 1) provide containment, 2) foster relationships, 3) promote emotional self-regulation, and 4) advance psychological recovery.

When clients with eating disorders are moving to a lower level of care, and then have weekly rehearsals alongside this transition, the resulting structure provides containment by offering peer-led meal support. Additionally, since people were engaging in rehearsal – twice a week, in the case of this production – it was a motivating factor that helped participants to not engage with their eating disorder. Furthermore, the clear parameters set regarding the expectations of working recovery and being able to be in the production were reported as containing and motivating factors for recovery.

The CoATT Model's ability to foster relationships provided another major benefit. Participants noted that being in a theatrical production took a commitment to themselves, and more importantly to others, which created a positive feedback loop that supported building relationships. Most importantly, the transition from the treatment world to the recovered world meant building a new support network, and the friendships that were made during the project were deeply valuable in the transition.

Third, participants reported that being in a CoATT production allowed them to work on emotional self-regulation. They could regulate through metaphor rather than by using an eating disorder behavior. Additionally, they shared that the process allowed them to get out of their comfort zone with an increased window of tolerance built by being in the production. The "window of tolerance" concept (Siegel, 1999) posits that people can take more risks in the world at large as they develop a higher tolerance for emotional discomfort.

Finally, participants revealed several ways in which their psychological recovery was advanced through the CoATT process. Unfinished business that did not get fully worked through in higher levels of care was explored. For example, one participant worked through issues of anger and the relationship with her mother in the final scene. Cognitive distortions were challenged as participants encountered an audience giving real-time feedback.

Another way that participants addressed psychological recovery was by learning to take up space in performance. An eating disorder often reinforces messages of being small, shutting down needs, and disappearing. Being in a CoATT production challenged those thought processes and allowed participants to feel seen and witnessed.

Participants expressed their connection to authenticity. One reason individuals fear giving up their eating disorder is because they do not know who their authentic self is underneath or outside of the disorder. Individuals with eating disorders worry that if the mask of the eating disorder is pulled back there will be nothing underneath. The eating disorder has become all-consuming, leaving clients not knowing who they are or what they like in the world. The process of developing authenticity is essential in the recovery process. Participants said that being in the CoATT process allowed them to shift the relationship they have with their bodies. Theatre, with its inherent focus on embodiment, allows clients to renegotiate the relationship and appreciation they have for their bodies. When scenes with highly physical action and expression are written into the play the benefits are palpable.

Overall, participants stated that the CoATT structure allowed them to enroll as agents of change in the community. As participants engage with the audience after performing a play focused on working through themes of recovery, they are witnessed and seen as experts by the audience. This is particularly salient for audience members who are working on their own recovery. As Callie shared in her post-process interview: "I've talked to so many people since the play that are, like, really identifying with this. I had people Facebook messaging me, being like, I don't know you, but can we meet for coffee because I really want to talk to you about how this play affected me." (Wood, 2016 p. 152). These results not only corroborated many areas that Noordenboors (2011a) spoke to regarding comprehensive recovery, but they also aligned with Herman's (2015) notion of reconnection as a necessity for transformation.

Finally, as a part of the launch process, participants created a group poem as a transitional object. They also kept meaningful props or costume pieces as a reminder of this step in their journey. The text of their poem highlights many aspects of their shared experience.

ACT ONE

I didn't think I was capable
Of doing something different
It's not that easy
It's not that easy
Doing the same thing over
and over
Again
You have to experience before judging

A look into
my Head (doubt)
Feelings (faith)
Heart (doubt)
Fear.

ACT TWO

I didn't want to let the production down
(We wanted people to understand)
You've got to be the real you
(Is the world ready to hear?)
Fear is a big thing

Let go
Let the play happen
Fear goes out the window

You can't mess up the lines when you wrote them

(Fear goes out the window)

The play came and rescued me.

ACT THREE

I remember
The hairs on the back of my neck dancing and tingling
(dancing and tingling)

An unexplainable joy
To touch someone's emotions (They understood)

Holding me accountable
Fighting to have good relationships with others
Watching people grow in difficult ways
Transforming myself
A part of my recovery I'll never forget

                    They understood.

                        Now
          I have faith that something can work
            The best recovery is living

A lengthier discussion of the study, including additional details, can be found in Wood (2016).

Conclusion

CoATT answers a very real call to eating disorder treatment but does not serve as a standalone treatment. Responses from participants of *Twin Falls* asserted that CoATT is particularly unique and is distinct from talk therapy given the way the CoATT model specifically paralleled experiences unique to recovery. It offered participants a touchstone experience to call back upon as they worked toward their recovery in the world at large. The medicine is written into the script, providing tangible lines and lessons to recall and apply in the here and now. As one participant beautifully summarized: "Now, every time I go into a therapy session, I can be, like, 'I'm going to feel this and I'm going to be fine when I leave and feel better about it.' It was so good, like, can we do the play every day? I never imagined I would have grown so much from doing the play. I never imagined ... I would be thinking about my character and what the next right thing for her would be or thinking about the play and everything it taught me. It's, like, part of my story in my recovery, in my life, in my perception" (Wood, 2016 p. 156).

    We imagine a world where partial and intensive outpatient eating disorder treatment centers partner with a CoATT team, and the process is used as a clear part of a transition plan. This allows for a greater connection, a sustained recovery, and a meaningful cycle for individuals who will be stepping down in their care. Individuals in treatment centers would have the opportunity to witness the production and then, themselves, be a part of the next round offered. A virtual cycle of connection, reconnection, and reinforced bonds to a community of others who value the experience and perspective of all who are working to maintain recovery, may reverse the cycle of relapse and re-hospitalization.

Reference List

American Psychiatric Association, D. S. M. T. F., & American Psychiatric Association. (2013). *Diagnostic and statistical manual of mental disorders: DSM-5* (Vol. 5, No. 5). Washington, DC: American psychiatric association. (5th ed.). 10.1176/appi.books.9780890425596.

Glaser, B., & Strauss, A. (2017). *Discovery of grounded theory: Strategies for qualitative research*. Routledge.

Herman, J. (2015). *Trauma and recovery*. Basic Books.

Jones, C., Harris, G., & Leung, N. (2005). Core beliefs and eating disorder recovery. *European Eating Disorders Review: The Professional Journal of the Eating Disorders Association, 13*(4): 237–244.

Marinilli Pinto, A., Guarda, A. S., Heinberg, L. J., & DiClemente, C. C. (2006). Development of the eating disorder recovery self-efficacy questionnaire. *International Journal of Eating Disorders, 39*(5): 376–384. 10.1002/eat.20256

Moore, M. (2015, May 22). *Only hope* [Video]. YouTube. https://www.youtube.com/watch?v=NTQBf06rboE

Noordenbos, G. (2011a). When have eating disordered patients recovered and what do the DSM-IV criteria tell about recovery? *Eating Disorders, 19*(3): 234–245. 10.1080/10640266.2011.564979

Noordenbos, G. (2011b). Which criteria for recovery are relevant according to eating disorder patients and therapists? *Eating Disorders, 19*(5): 441–451. 10.1080/10640266.2011.618738

Siegel, D. J. (1999). *The developing mind: Toward a neurobiology of interpersonal experience.* Guilford.

Wilson, G. T., Grilo, C. M., & Vitousek, K. M. (2007). Psychological treatment of eating disorders. *The American Psychologist, 62*(3): 199–216. 10.1037/0003-066X.62.3.199

Wonderlich, S., Mitchell, J. E., Crosby, R. D., Myers, T. C., Kadlec, K., LaHaise, K., Swan-Kremeier, L., Dokken, J., Lange, M., Dinkel, J., Jorgensen, M., & Schnader, L. (2012). Minimizing and treating chronicity in eating disorders: A clinical overview. *The International Journal of Eating Disorders, 45*(4): 467–475. 10.1002/eat.20978

Wood, L. L. (2016). *The use of therapeutic theater in supporting clients in eating disorder recovery after intensive treatment: A qualitative study* [Doctoral dissertation, University of Missouri, St. Louis]. UMSL Libraries. https://irl.umsl.edu/dissertation/21

Wood, L. L., Hartung, S., Al-Qadfan, F., Wichmann, S., Cho, A. B., & Bryant, D. (2022). Drama therapy and the treatment of eating disorders: Advancing towards clinical guidelines. *The Arts in Psychotherapy, 80*: Article 101948. 10.1016/j.aip.2022.101948

Chapter 6

Aphasia Recovery

Introduction

CoATT scripts built by and for people living with aphasia reflect the ways in which CoATT manualization can be easily adapted for a unique recovery population. The script for *The Gift* demonstrates a structure that both supports treatment goals for participants working on speech goals *and* opens into thematic and personal material that furthers psycho-social goals for participants. The discipline needed to adapt the model for participants living with aphasia pays off with a powerful co-active audience participation piece that focuses on both elements of treatment. Impressive progress on speech is made more poignant and relevant when it focuses on themes that matter: family, parenting, and the connections that make meaning in our lives.

Aphasia

Aphasia is an acquired language disorder that causes damage to the brain, most often due to stroke. Aphasia typically results in deficits in multiple domains, including speech and comprehension, as well as in reading and writing. Despite these language challenges, persons with aphasia are otherwise highly functioning and typically do not have an intellectual disability because of their aphasia.

Aphasia affects approximately 2 million people in the United States, and, although aphasia is a common diagnosis, approximately 84.5 percent of people cannot identify or describe the disorder (National Aphasia Alliance). The frequent misconceptions and general lack of understanding about aphasia have important effects on both the social-emotional and practical aspects of persons with aphasia. Practically, misconceptions about the disorder often leave people with aphasia avoiding communication with others, resulting in language skills that remain the same as their post-stroke baseline (Dalemans et al., 2010). When language skills do not improve, an aphasic individual's social-emotional wellness may suffer, leaving many persons with aphasia fearful of being judged, left out, or experiencing a sense of loss

DOI: 10.4324/9781003161608-7

regarding their former identity (Cruice et al., 2003). On the more acute end, aphasia can result in individuals feeling isolated, anxious, or depressed (Code & Herrmann, 2003).

Treatment as Usual

Typical treatment of aphasia focuses on the recovery of language skills, including comprehension, expression, reading, and writing, which are specifically in service of promoting participation in society (Ross & Wertz, 2003). Persons with aphasia typically attend regular weekly speech-language therapy sessions. Simmons-Mackie and Damico (2011) asserted that emotional and psychological issues are present during speech-language pathology sessions, and, while counseling is considered within the scope of practice for speech-language pathologists, clinicians regularly avoid approaching these topics in a meaningful way due to professional values, or a lack of clinical training and capacity to sit with and tolerate difficult emotions. Therefore, if the primary focus of sessions remains fact- and skill-based, and traditional talk therapy becomes inaccessible, persons with aphasia are left with few professional options for processing and exploring the complex emotions resulting from their aphasia.

Aphasia Recovery

Aphasia recovery has primarily been operationalized by professionals as the recovery of language and evaluated based on psychometric assessments. Although language is the primary factor that dictates aphasia recovery, some scholars argue that considering a more holistic approach to recovery could be beneficial for the operationalization of aphasia recovery. This includes non-linguistic factors and their impact on neural networks (Cahana-Amitay & Albert, 2015) but can also include a multilevel framework that considers the complex interrelation between neural, cognitive, and behavioral aspects (Code, 2001).

As previously mentioned, even though there are studies on the social-emotional impact of aphasia, and the correlation between mental wellness and linguistic recovery, the social-emotional needs of aphasia patients are not formally considered a part of recovery. In a qualitative study of persons with aphasia and their experiences of social-emotional wellness conducted by Dalemans et al. (2010), persons with aphasia reported feeling "burdensome to others and wish to function in an ordinary way ... often they are not able to work, and they wish to contribute to the community in other ways. Although they often feel stigmatized, they wish to be respected. Often, they do not reach that goal" (p. 537). The medical model does not formally include social-emotional factors as primary to aphasia recovery, persons with aphasia themselves may very well see these aspects as a crucial part of their recovery. Therefore, finding unique ways to honor their recovery as they see it is essential. CoATT can provide an original avenue that addresses formal definitions of aphasia recovery by targeting language goals while also empowering aphasic individuals to narrate what will benefit their recovery.

Considerations with CoATT and Aphasia

When we initially conceptualized the CoATT model, we knew it was a recovery-focused model, but our primary recovery populations at the time were clients with eating disorders, trauma, and substance use disorders. While presenting at a university conference on the model we were approached by the speech-language team at the institution. They were convinced that the model could also be applicable to persons with aphasia. So we cracked open textbooks and learned about aphasia while working very closely with the speech-language team to understand the unique needs of the population. This practice is in line with our model in that later, at every rehearsal, a speech-language therapist would be present, serving as the population specialist for the group.

Aphasia places real strains on participants in the CoATT model, so modifications are needed. Some adaptations are straightforward: we make sessions slightly longer (2.5 hours), which include rest and snack breaks; we limit the time of the Intensive movement to half days; and we have interns to support participants with the homework, which is done after a session or in individual speech-language sessions.

The other major modification was the addition of clear speech/language goals, as dictated by the speech-language pathology team. The team gave each individual baseline language evaluations and made recommended goals in conjunction with their individual therapy. For example, these goals included increasing sentence utterance, such as going from three-word sentences to four or including words with challenging pronunciations.

Production: The Gift

The Gift included cast members who had previous experience with the CoATT model. They brought wisdom to the process, as well as an advanced understanding and long-term experience with recovery into the sessions. In addition to speech therapy goals, the psychosocial goals are identified by CP1 and are offered to CP2 so that they can suggest an arc for each character. For the play to work, each beat and each scene must move the story forward. Given the limitations on speech, we find that each line must work to advance the journey of each character. By assigning a simple character arc that reflects both speech goals and psychosocial growth, the script supports breakthroughs in both areas.

Participants

Before we even start writing the story and pulling together a script, we're looking for clues to indicate the structure we will need. Here, it helped to have a clear plan for each of our actors.

Gayle came to the group with an advanced understanding of recovery and strong experience working in the model. She had an expanded capacity for speaking and enjoyed performing. She successfully performed in a large role for her first CoATT production, *Aphasia Park*. Her goals included maintaining control of speech in moments of emotion, and more fluidity with conversational patterns.

Brett was the only male in the group and was several years into his recovery. In the previous play, Brett developed the role of "the Entertainer," and he was confident in his musical and comedic abilities. His goals included playing a larger role and initiating exchanges.

Pamela returned to the group with high energy, enormous presence and personality, and self-deprecating humor that masked her struggles with memory and speech. Her goal was to perform with less need for support, in terms of both prompting for lines and physical tasks.

Aleta was also a veteran of the first round. Her speech was limited to one word at a time, she was physically unsteady due to the residual effects of the stroke, and she required assistance to participate in rehearsal. Her needs were easy to accommodate with support provided by her aide or by an intern in the speech program. She succeeded in the group through force of will and dedication, bringing an easy smile and an untiring spirit. In the previous CoATT experience, her caregivers and support network struggled to embrace the process, worrying that it would be "too challenging," or would prove to be "embarrassing." After her resounding success, she joined the second group with goal of increasing her word count and having more interaction with other ensemble members.

Tonia was a new member of the group. The speech team, supportive of the CoATT experience, cleared her for participation. Socialization with peers, sustained concentration, and the opportunity to increase spontaneity in vocalization were the stated goals of her participation.

For *The Gift*, the second and third movements of the CoATT model yielded key elements of the final script and presentation. The basic script emerged from the earliest meetings, giving time for the participants to deliver a strong presentation of a well-made play while continuing to improvise, refine, and pursue both angles of their therapy. The basic script needed to be structured to meet the limitations of the participants' language, stamina, and physical abilities. It had to be built to be achievable through repetition and practice. Both stage directions and dialogue were concrete and detailed so that all members of the staff and cast could visualize, rehearse, and remember the play for a successful presentation.

Excerpt and Commentary

In the first group meeting, CP1 followed the manualized exercise, "Play your recovery," and in an adaptation of this exercise invited the group to play recovery as a team. Given this, there are two important reasons for working as a group. First, the element of time: Since speech is slow and the exercise must unfold during the session, working in groups is simply more efficient. Secondly, the group is forming its own definition of "recovery from aphasia." As noted above, the medical model cannot provide one standard definition of recovery for people with an aphasia diagnosis. Rather, each individual may reach a level of recovery that is dependent upon their symptoms. Therefore, each particular group works around the concept of recovery to describe what it is like for them at the time of the production.

The theme that emerged in this round of exploration was "slow." Here, there is an answer to the CoATT model prompt: What is one thing you want the audience to know about recovery? In various ways, each group member described recovery as "slow." This included self-descriptions such as "I talk slow now," and "I need time to communicate." It also served as a reflection on the process of recovery, as in "My recovery is slow, but I'm doing the best that I can," and "I may need you to be patient with me" or "I know I am slow, but please don't finish my sentences for me."

The discussion turned to the way in which society values speed, and the actual rate at which information and activity happens. The group acknowledged that recovery from aphasia takes time, but also agreed that the pace of society does not allow recovery to unfold. In this way, the group stated that recovery from aphasia should be given the time it needs. This live issue elicited responses that not only defined recovery for the group, but also shaped the theme of the play: As a result of our recovery, we value going slow.

In the third week, as scene work began, another adaptation allowed the group to work efficiently toward a concrete script. While still working as an ensemble, the group explored three key prompts. First, CP1 prepared stories that presented speed, and an exercise that explored both speed and its opposite, "slow." Second, CP1 led improvisation and monologue work using "The Tortoise and the Hare," and then moved into a physical group improvisation. Relying less on speech but pushing against some physical limitations created by brain injury, the group created "machines." These sculpts required that the entire ensemble be connected to each other, and that the physical tasks each person chose influenced the others. In movement, these sculpts held the cast together through sequence, rhythm, eye contact, and, sometimes, through physical connections. Most importantly, the machine sculptures allowed the group to work together, whether going fast or slowing down. This exercise physically illustrated what it means to "slow down for each other" or to "help each other go more quickly." When the message of the group to its audience is limited in verbal expression, the illustration becomes even more important.

Another session used a butterfly story that resonated deeply with the group. They were emotional as they embodied the stages of butterfly development. We used a story resembling the following:

A man spent hours watching a butterfly struggling to emerge from its cocoon. [The butterfly] managed to make a small hole, but its body was too large to get through it. After a long struggle, it appeared to be exhausted and remained absolutely still.

The man decided to help the butterfly and, with a pair of scissors, he cut open the cocoon, thus releasing the butterfly. However, the butterfly's body was very small and wrinkled and its wings were all crumpled.

The man continued to watch, hoping that, at any moment, the butterfly would open its wings and fly away. Nothing happened; in fact, the butterfly spent the rest of its brief life dragging around its shrunken body and shrivelled wings, incapable of flight.

What the man – out of kindness and his eagerness to help – had failed to understand was that the tight cocoon and the efforts that the butterfly had to make in order to squeeze out of that tiny hole were Nature's way of training the butterfly and of strengthening its wing.

Sometimes, a little extra effort is precisely what prepares us for the next obstacle to be faced. Anyone who refuses to make that effort, or gets the wrong sort of help, is left unprepared to fight the next battle and never manages to fly off to their destiny. (Coelho, 2007)

Acting out this long piece of text was exhausting. As each beat of the story unfolded, decisions about how to present the imagery were handled by the group. Who will be the boy? Who will be the caterpillar? How can we use all of us to create a theatrical image or sculpt to show the stages of development? The work on machines had yielded more than the theme of "fast/slow." It developed the kinetic awareness of the group and refined their ability to work together. Again, this group was preparing to communicate with an audience about their wisdom in recovery. The stage pictures are one way to say, "Let us show you what we mean."

The simple story with an agonizing twist resembles Augusto Boal's childhood story of helping chicks break out of their shells in the farmyard, only for them to die in harsh conditions. The similarity in prompts is a reminder of the underlying ethos of *Theater of the Oppressed* (Boal, 1974); where the spectator becomes the spectator, providing an opportunity for the group to work through an unanswered question and determine their own resolution. Such stories often contain the wisdom of the imperfect solution or the pointless intervention. The group was satisfied with the butterfly metaphor and insisted on incorporating the passage. They found a metaphor that worked for them, focused on the positive aspect of supported transformation and ignoring the twist. This is a reminder that CP1 and CP2 should both be prepared to suggest stories or incorporate prompts that have proven meaningful in previous experiences when it comes to scene work in the generation phase.

Writing the script for *The Gift,* therefore, began with several strong anchor points. The theme was clear: "We value going slow as a result of our recovery." There were two anchor images: "As a group we will portray the development of a butterfly, and we can use the machine concept to illustrate slow and fast. We also have requirements for our ensemble members, such as Brett will play the piano and entertain us with a song. Any play we write will have to include these elements."

What else did we know as we prepared to make the script for *The Gift?* We knew that we needed to juxtapose traditional narrative with the magical poetic imagery of an ensemble portraying a butterfly. We knew that there were limits to the movement and speech of the actors, and we knew that the stage directions would have to be concrete and detailed in order to help with execution. For these reasons, we chose to construct the story as a "memory play." The conventions of a story like this one allow a narrator to speak in a way that helps to set the story efficiently and to move the action forward through language. Memory is never exact; it lends itself to the blend of realism and theatricality. This combination is what our "set pieces" like the butterfly sequence require in order to make sense for an audience. Memory plays also allow us to put our support people (in this case, an intern from the speech pathology program) on stage with the performers to handle larger sections of text while simultaneously aiding in the physical demands of the performance. This can look like possibly steadying the balance of an ensemble member, carrying a prop, or assisting in an exit and transition.

A close reading of the script suggests that these requirements came together easily and created a very straightforward story. While it is surprising to imagine that a laundry list of boundaries, restrictions, and set pieces make it easier to find a narrative throughline, this is a backbone concept in the manualization of the CoATT model. The early movements yield insight and direction, as well as text and staging, for the script presented at the end of the Intensive. *The Gift*, as a working script, shows the way co-active creation delivers on the therapeutic goals of the group.

THE GIFT

<u>CAST OF CHARACTERS</u> **(1)**

ABIGAIL (a teenager) . . . . .Danielle
Her AUNT PENNY. . . . . .Pamela
Her mother, GLENDA. . . . . .Gale
Her father, BEN. . . . . .Brett
Her AUNT AMY. . . . . .Aleta
Her AUNT TILLY. . . . . .Tonya

<u>Setting</u>

A family room on Long Island. There's a couch and coffee
table. A comfortable chair corners the set a little down
left. Down right is a piano, with a bench. The piano shows
where the wall is by running straight up stage, if you sit
there you are in profile to the audience. There is a door that
leads to the rest of the house just upstage of the piano. Out
that door would be a hallway to three bedrooms. ABIGAIL, the
teenage daughter and only child, has a room that is all the way
at the end of the hall. Upstage left in the corner of the stage
is the front door, opening outside. So the upstage wall has a
window. In the downstage left corner, directly opposite the
piano is a door to the kitchen **(2)**

This is a memory play. Abigail is remembering her 15th
birthday. So the house isn't solid with walls. Maybe there's
nothing outside the window. Maybe she is telling us about a
scene that she wasn't actually there for . . . but it's how she
imagines it might go. What we see is just what ABIGAIL re-
members. For example, as the lights come up, she is standing
by the kitchen door, downstage left. Behind her is her
family lined up in a freeze position, a line with her AUNT
PENNY, her mother GLENDA, her father BEN, her AUNT AMY, and
her AUNT TILLY.

1 Even the cast list provides evidence for how the concrete and detailed first draft of the play reflects the group. Notice that each character has a name that reflects the participant, which provides ease when scanning a script, and familiarity. While it may seem like an obvious way to name characters, it stands in contrast to the way other character names evolve in the CoATT model. Here, the CP2 names the character for "ease of use," while in most other creative processes, the cast themselves would name characters as part of the expressive exploration in early movements. Danielle, the speech pathology intern, gets an unrelated character name, one chosen by her in the rehearsal process.

2 Concrete stage directions allow participants to imagine, remember, or practice the play on their own time. This is followed by an introduction to the concept of "memory play." It is included in the script to support the participants in acting the scenes as written. When much of the work centers on concrete measurement of progress toward goals, it's important to give a rationale for anything that steers the participant into less certain territory. Additionally, since we teach acting as behaving "truthfully in imaginary situations" (Meisner, 1987, p. 15), we are careful to provide reality-based descriptions alongside any imaginary cues. The best examples of this thinking are the description of imaginary walls, written to explain why we don't have a set on hand, and the explanation that the narrator might be aware of scenes in which she does not appear. A shared understanding of the logic of the play is important to the success of the ensemble, just as important as a shared understanding of the recovery concept is, as well. The description of the opening tableau serves two purposes. First, it minimizes the need for physical entrance and exit, and second, it sets up the "machine that goes faster or slower," which was taken from the earlier movements in the CoATT model.

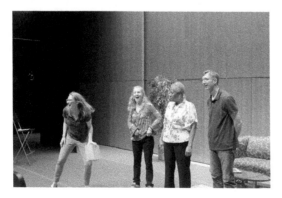

Figure 6.1 Dr. Wood meets with the cast in rehearsal. Photograph by Sarah Martin (@sleepypaints).

ABIGAIL
(ABIGAIL talks directly to the audience) **(3)**
I am an only child, but I come from a big family. I have
three Aunties who were always at our house. Aunt Penny is
my Dad's sister. That is her at the front of the line. My
mom, Glenda and dad, BEN, always invited them to our
house. There is my mom's sisters, Aunt Amy and Aunt Tilly.
They always made a big deal about my birthday, gave me a lot
of presents. But the year I turned 15 I was a typical
teenager. I wanted to have a party with my friends. I did
not want to stay home with my family. I was impatient to be
a grownup and have all the answers. Little did I know, the
year I turned 15 I was going to get a very special gift ...

(She exits out the door to her room.)

(The lights shift to show the family room. The adults
are wrapping gifts. It is like a GIFT MACHINE.) **(4)**

AUNT PENNY
Box!

GLENDA
Gift!

BEN
Wrap!

AUNT AMY
Bow!

AUNT TILLY
Love it!

AUNT PENNY
Box!

GLENDA
Gift!

BEN
Wrap!

AUNT AMY
Bow!

3   The character of Abigail, played by an intern, drives the narrative of this story and drives the action on the stage. Her narrative sets up the relationships of the play, and her character will undergo the change that illustrates the group's message. Describing herself as a typical teenager, she says, "I was impatient to be a grownup and have all the answers." Our play starts by locating the premise in a dramatic arc, placing the character as far away from the wisdom she will gain as possible. Each line and each scene will move her closer to the understanding that our participants hope the audience will share: "as a result of our recovery, we value going slow."

4   Upon her exit, the characters launch the "machine" that had been explored. The script sets up a sequence of lines and actions that can repeat, the way a machine performs a repetitive task. We move through one round of the actions called "Box. Gift. Wrap. Bow. Love it!" This sequence could be sped up or slowed down. The intention behind this set piece was to repeat it for comic effect, exaggerating the speed and execution of the sequence as a comic way to underline the speed that the participants struggle with in life. The repetition proved too difficult, though, so instead, the script includes an interruption by Abigail, which makes her responsible for creating the rush. As the pattern gets shorter, the same comic energy is found as long as the actors use each line to interact with each other.

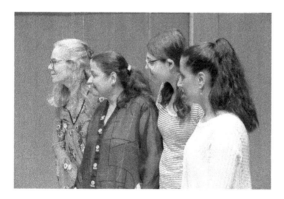

Figure 6.2 Abigail's aunties are concerned. Photograph by Sarah Martin (@sleepypaints).

(This time ABIGAIL comes in from her room and just grabs the almost finished gift from AUNT AMY.)

ABIGAIL

Is this for me?! Awesome.

(She exits into the kitchen.)

AUNT PENNY

Box!

GLENDA

Gift!

BEN

Wrap!

(ABIGAIL comes back in headed to her room. She interrupts her dad.)

ABIGAIL

Oh cool! Dad! Thanks you guys.

(So they start one more time)

AUNT PENNY

Box!

GLENDA

Gift!

(ABIGAIL comes back in. She interrupts her mother.)

ABIGAIL

You guys, technically my birthday is tomorrow.

(The AUNTIES are just shocked. And GLENDA is embarrassed.) **(5)**

GLENDA

No. Wait a minute. You need to be more polite.

ABIGAIL

Sorry, Mom. But those were for me anyways, right?

5 Abigail is portrayed as a typical teenager, but it was important to demonstrate that she wasn't badly behaved or motivated by hostility or greed. The participants wanted to explore the challenges of being in a family, of parenting, of navigating the process that others are going through while facing the challenges and limitations of their aphasia. Participants in our aphasia group continue to develop the script through the rehearsal process, as do all CoATT groups. The extended discussions that usually take longer due to the group's rate of speech yield more reflection (and rewriting) than those in other CoATT groups. Abigail's speech was one point on which reflection often centered. Our participants were eager to show that they understood the point of view of younger characters. For them, this was part of being a good parent, but also part of demonstrating that their parenting skills were "intact" behind the aphasia.

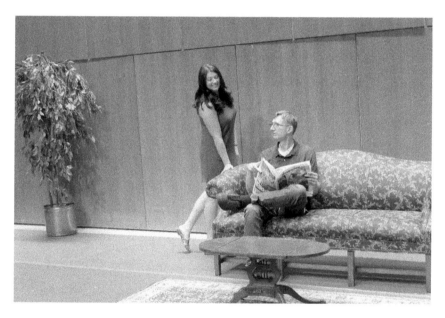

Figure 6.3 A teenage daughter engages in a conversation with her father. Photograph by Sarah Martin (@sleepypaints).

                    GLENDA
Yes. But you need to learn to wait. Not everything happens on your time. **(6)**

                    ABIGAIL
Mom, gosh. It's not that big a deal.

                    GLENDA
Yes it is. If you are always interrupting, you might miss
part of the gift.

                    ABIGAIL
Mom!

                    GLENDA
Don't talk back to me. You're grounded for the weekend.

        (ABIGAIL storms off to her bedroom.)

                  AUNT TILLY
Our niece is having a hard time lately.

                  AUNT PENNY
        She is. She is rushing everywhere.

                   AUNT AMY
Rushing. Always rushing. **(7)**

                  AUNT TILLY
Let's go in the kitchen - we could use a break.

                  AUNT PENNY
Good idea. We can brainstorm how to help her.

                   AUNT AMY
Yes. Good idea. Let's go.

        (GLENDA and the AUNTIES walk into the kitchen.)

6   Even the act of rehearsing and developing the speech for Abigail underlined the key theme for the group: "It may be slower to work with us, but there is wisdom and value in going slower." Participant G, as Glenda, drops three pieces of powerful parenting into her next three lines: "You need to be polite," "Everything doesn't 'happen on your time,'" and "You might miss part of the gift." The scene allowed for reflections on parenting between participants, most of whom were parenting children at home. They agreed, as most parents would, that getting through to a teenager with one good piece of advice would be a victory! Abigail, though, like most teens, isn't listening as closely as her mother might wish. So, Glenda must show another strong parenting technique: she sets a boundary and Abigail is grounded.

7   The short speech that motivates the exit of the Aunties contained the first speech goal for Participant Aleta. Aunt Amy says, "Rushing. Always rushing." It is the first sentence that this participant has performed with more than one word in it. In previous productions, her character had one word that was spoken toward the end of the play: the repeated word, "painting." So, with this sentence, our participant has spoken two sentences and has added a second word into the "demand" of her lines. Crucially, this line flows with the dialogue of the others, and therefore, is subject to the "speed of the machine." With one line, Participant Aleta has dramatized her wisdom from recovery. For the other two Aunties, the lines contain concrete stage directions, which allow them to tie in speech with action, and increase the likelihood that they will recall the proper line. For Participant Pamela, playing Aunt Penny decreased her focus on remembering the correct word and lessened the pressure on her speech. It allowed her to connect the impulse to the move, to take the next logical action and to use her speech as a natural expression of the moment. Consider that Glenda is not presented as a "parent with aphasia," nor does Abigail treat her mother as diminished in any way. We're presented with a scene that any parent might benefit from witnessing: a dramatization of teenage speed and how challenging it can be for a parent. The archetypal presentation of these family roles builds through the next sequences, driven by our all-too-familiar team.

ABIGAIL

Can I talk to you Dad? **(8)**

BEN

Sure.

ABIGAIL

I can't be grounded this weekend. I want to have my birthday party with my friends.

BEN

Well, I think you have to stay home. You're grounded.

ABIGAIL

But that's not fair. I said I was sorry. And I can have a party with you any time. This is with my friends.

BEN

I understand.

ABIGAIL

You do. I knew you would. So I can go?

BEN

You better ask your mother.

(GLENDA comes in from the kitchen.)

ABIGAIL

Dad says I can go to a birthday party with my friends this weekend.

GLENDA

No, you cannot. You are grounded.

ABIGAIL

Dad said I could! **(9)**

BEN

I said I understand your feelings. But I did not say you could go.

GLENDA

That's right. There is an important lesson to be learned here.

BETTY

Dad! You said!

8   The intern playing Abigail found herself in the middle of the discussion when this scene was in rehearsal. The participants had lots of advice for her and offered many rounds of direction on how to play the character. Including this scene benefited the group by providing a prompt for psychosocial interaction, by the building of the bonds of respect, and by the opportunities for sharing a wide variety of experiences and points of view on family behavior. This easy interaction is noted in the results of the study that are attached to the CoATT production. Abigail finds herself alone with her father, Ben, and tries to manipulate the situation to her advantage. This scene reveals an emotional intelligence in Ben; he dramatizes for us, again, that a depth of understanding bubbles under a quiet surface of limited linguistic expression. His daughter is secure enough with him to show her real frustration and her inner desires, and he truly does understand her. He also understands the contract of parenting between partners; he will back up his wife and hold the boundary. Admirably, he will not speak on behalf of Glenda. He sends Abigail straight back to her and suggests that the two of them resolve the conflict.

9   Our teen protagonist twists his words ever so slightly, saying, "Dad said I could go," but Ben corrects her with clarity and specificity about the exact words he spoke to her. This typical exchange, in which a child attempts to play one parent against another, is a powerful moment that carried deep meaning for our participants. Again, the scene returns to a parenting concern and presents useful wisdom and healthy modeling. These are good parents, undiminished by their aphasia. Again, the play demonstrates that our participants understand everything going on around them, whether they are verbose or not. Further, the script shows how important words are, and how much more specific and powerful they become when they must be chosen slowly and carefully. Ben is able to be a good father and a good husband with careful consideration of his speech. In fact, his behavior in the scene dramatizes the importance of slowing down when dealing with those we love.

                         BEN
No. I said we should speak to your mother. I agree
with her.

                         BETTY
Ugh. I just want to go out.

        (BETTY goes to the bedroom.)

                        GLENDA
We have to stick together.

                         BEN
We will. We are a team.

                        GLENDA
I don't want her to miss out on this part of life.

                         Ben
I know. None of us do. **(10)**

   (The AUNTIES poke their heads in.)

                      AUNT TILLY
Is it okay for us to come in?

                      AUNT PENNY
We were feeling worried.

                        GLENDA
We want her to be with us for her birthday. I want her to
slow down and enjoy her family.

                      AUNT TILLY
She is upset to be grounded ... but she was being so rude!

                         BEN
I know. It's hard to be a teenager. Maybe we can teach her
about compromise. Let's have a surprise party for her now
and then she can have time for her friends later this
weekend too. **(11)**

                      AUNT AMY
Let's get balloons!

                         ALL
Yes. Balloons.

10   Despite ample opportunity for the group to reflect on this short scene during the Rehearsal movement, there was very little rewriting. Even though it went unspoken, the action of the scene underlines the competence of people living with aphasia; just because they have some impaired communication, that does not make them easy marks for manipulation. One theme mentioned early in the Generation movement stated this concern more bluntly: "Don't think we are stupid just because we talk this way." The participants seemed satisfied that this brief scene demonstrated the theme adequately.

CoATT-model plays are aimed at a public audience, and construction of these plays is meant to facilitate the most powerful performances possible. Audiences come expecting to see good acting and to see scenes that feel relevant, truthful, and emotionally charged, which is exactly what they might expect from any play at any theatre. This becomes a guiding principle for participants as they create characters and approach scenes. From this, the scripts contain real conflict and emotional content. So, when reflecting on the scenes, the actors might be aligned around themes and the messages embedded in the script. The onstage characters are strongly motivated by individual points of view and are pressured by their imaginary circumstances.

11   Ben turns to his wife at an interesting moment, having just united with her on an action that is bound to upset their teenager. This realistic pressure is met with an odd, but understandable impulse: the need for compromise. He offers a creative solution, a reasonable compromise that might help maintain the boundary, but still celebrate as a family. This impulse comes directly from Participant Brett, who plays Ben. This storytelling decision received unanimous ratification by the entire cast. Hence, the offer to throw a party for the badly behaved teen becomes the next part of the action on stage. It happens to support a goal for Participant B, offering a chance for the actor to present "the Entertainer" role and play the piano.

AUNT PENNY

I will go get the delicious food. All her favorites!

GLENDA

I will get the wine. For the grownups, of course! **(12)**

BEN

I can play the music!

(They go to the kitchen.)

AUNT TILLY

I will get the decorations ready. We can hang up streamers and a beautiful sign!

AUNT AMY

I'll help you!

(She goes behind the couch. There is a sign to hold up later: "Happy Birthday Abby" on flags, one letter each, on a clothesline with two poles. Two AUNTIES will hold it up later. Balloons should be pre-set and inflated.)

(GLENDA and AUNT PENNY return with cake and drinks. BEN goes to the piano.)

BEN

Maybe this song?

(They sing a little.)

AUNT TILLY

Shhh! She will hear us.

(They are laughing.)

(ABIGAIL does come in.)

GLENDA

What are you doing out of your room? We were trying to surprise you early so you could slow down and spend time with us and your friends.

ABIGAIL

Well, it's too late! You were too slow!

12 Abigail's comment is selfish and cruel, especially in the context of parents who have aphasia. But the impulse is very human and was important for the actor creating the role of Ben to work through in the performance. While the party seems to derail the engine of the plot (i.e., the conflict between teenager and parents), it is a realistic portrait of family dynamics, and while the party seems to move the message of the play away from the theme of "we value going slow," it offers an opportunity to raise the stakes for all the characters in the story. The clash between generations in a family often presents fast, jerky, and awkward exchanges. As the Aunties chime in, her mother, Glenda, feels the same pressure mounting. Participant Gale added a double-edged piece of humor to the moment with her comment, "I'll get the wine. For the adults." It diffuses some of the frustration, but also makes a key point that the participants tied to the theme in earlier discussions: "Don't treat us like children because of our condition." She's gone through the same repetition of frustrating conflict. Her daughter keeps behaving badly, no matter how she tries to help. Now, the family puts her in a compromising position with the party happening around her, and Abigail is still obstinate.

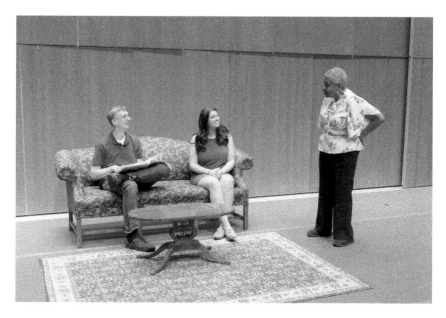

Figure 6.4 Two parents work to unite in their message for their teenage daughter. Photograph by Sarah Martin (@sleepypaints).

                    AUNTS AMY, TILLY, and PENNY
ABIGAIL!!!

> (They are together in front of the couch. The
> family begins to gather behind them.)

                    GLENDA
No. I want to tell you something. You are in a rush to grow
up, but everything takes its own time. A butterfly starts
as a caterpillar and goes into its cocoon. When the butterfly has made its transformation, it must come out of
the cocoon. If we were to rush up to the butterfly and pull
it out of its cocoon too soon, the butterfly would die. The
butterfly needs the process of coming out of the cocoon to
strengthen its wings so it can fly. **(13)**

> (A beat, she takes it in while the family builds
> the butterfly.) **(14)**

                    ABIGAIL
Oh ... now I get it.

> (Another beat.)

I'm sorry.

                    BEN
We are your family, and we are all here to help you learn
to slow down and take your time so you can truly fly.

                    AUNT PENNY
We have a gift for you, from all of us.

                    AUNT TILLY
Open it!

                    AUNT AMY
Open it!

> (While they are gathered around her, the box is
> opened and a silk scarf with butterflies on it
> comes out.)

13   Glenda has a monologue following this moment in the play. For any actor, a long monologue needs clear and compelling motivation. For an actor working with aphasia, however, there needs to be an especially high level of energy going into the speech. The risk, though, is that emotional pressure and conflict might derail the control she feels in managing a large chunk of language. Nevertheless, this is the task that is set up as a speech goal for Participant Gale. Her speech is cued by a direct set-up to the theme when Abigail says, "You were too slow!" Readers will notice that the monologue contains an abbreviated version of the "butterfly story" that was initially used as a prompt. This text serves the dual purpose of challenging Participant Gale with a long and emotionally charged leading actress moment while also moving the action toward the third "set piece" created by the group in the Generation movement. This speech was improvised many times during rehearsal, demonstrating both fluidity with language and risk-taking through the spoken relationship between Participant Gale and the intern playing Abigail.

14   The group built a movement piece to illustrate the same butterfly story, and they used a piece of silk as a prop to suggest wings. As the speech unfolds, and Abigail accepts the gift and lesson of the story, the group builds their sculpture around her. She is transformed into the image of a butterfly. The tableau serves as a beautiful and striking final image for the play and offers closure and comment through several dynamics.

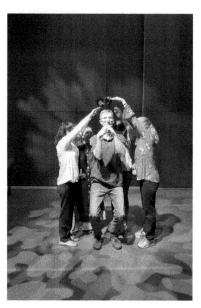

Figure 6.5 A family builds a butterfly cocoon to express a metaphorical story about "slowing down." Photograph by Sarah Martin (@sleepypaints).

(BEN goes to the piano. He plays Happy Birthday.
They all sing. He turns to his daughter.)

                    BEN
Make a wish!

(She takes a deep breath. The family is cocooned
around her. She blows out the candle and the stage
goes black.) **(15)**

(END OF PLAY) **(16)**

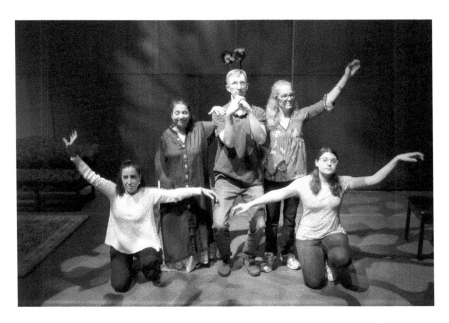

Figure 6.6 A family creates a tableau of a butterfly to accompany their metaphorical story about "slowing down." Photograph by Sarah Martin (@sleepypaints).

15 Notably, the final picture is independent of language; it is seen rather than spoken. The move away from the limitation that this group shares demonstrates one of the many strengths they bring to the creation of the play, as well as to recovery. They have learned to work together, more powerfully than they might have done on their own. By incorporating every player in the final sculpt, the full group endorses the theme and presentation of the play, and by demonstrating a slow building process that results in beauty, they are offering an explication of their theme. Just as Glenda's story suggests, the beauty is worth the wait.

16 The butterfly image extends the concept of recovery by conjuring the dynamic of transformation. And, in doing so, the group makes perhaps the wisest observation that they can offer to their audience, for it is not simply a self-centered plea for patience that underpins the advice to "slow down." Transformation is the demonstrated promise of recovery, illustrated through the theatrical metaphor of the butterfly; individuals are transformed into a group, and silk is transformed into wings, struggle into flow, and suffering into wisdom.

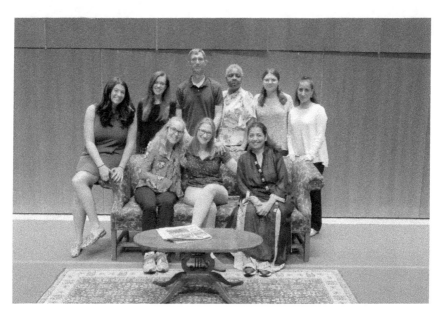

Figure 6.7 Photograph of the cast of The Gift. Photograph by Sarah Martin (@sleepy-paints).

The CoATT Interactive Element

Participants decided that the CoActive element they wanted to design for the audience was asking people to reflect on the things in their lives that helped them to slow down. It was their hope that providing this type of reflection for an audience would help deconstruct the dominant narrative privileging the fast-paced and fully able-bodied, and make room for the less-dominant narrative.

Audience members were provided index cards and asked to write down words, phrases, or advice about slowing down. The cards were then collected in a basket and were brought up by the participants. Participants drew cards and spontaneously read aloud the answers people provided (this became a very proud moment for cast members who were getting to show off their language skills in the moment, unrehearsed!). The phrases were then written down into a community poem, which was read back to the audience.

Results

Several measurements were conducted on the participants of *The Gift*. At the time of this book, two article publications were in process. The first examined the quantitative measures of speech-language improvement, and early data indicates positive trends. The second explored caregiver responses to the work. They reported that the greatest benefits for their loved ones with aphasia were making new friends, gaining confidence, feeling supported, and becoming more outgoing (Alimonti et al., in press). That aligns neatly with a previous study using the CoATT model with persons with aphasia (Wood et al., 2020), in which a qualitative focus group spotlighted the benefits of the CoATT model – including the opportunity to build meaningful relationships and improvement in speech-language abilities. Finally, a study on audience benefit was also conducted, finding ($n = 56$) that 77 percent of the surveyed audience members felt their knowledge and understanding of aphasia had increased. Additionally, during the interactive CoActive element, audience members were asked to write their feelings during and after the performance. Responses included: "Proud and inspired! "Reminds me why I am a speech therapist," and "I feel empathy." (Datta et al., in press)

Conclusion

The Gift illustrates several key elements of the CoATT model. First, the group shares their concept of recovery, defining it as a transformation. Second, the script uses that metaphor to explore the key theme of personal transformations: "We value going slow." Third, the script presents that theme through recognizable challenges that an audience can easily understand and relate to their own experiences. Their theme, which is the wisdom they choose to share in their new role as people recovering from brain injury and aphasia, is useful to teenagers and their parents in any average family dynamic.

The presentation of *The Gift* dramatizes recovery for the audience without limiting the experience to those with a previous understanding of aphasia. The CoATT process had to be adapted with just such a familiarity, though. Expertise in the challenges specific to people living with aphasia led to a carefully crafted script that moves both actor and idea forward with every word spoken. The CoATT model easily expands to allow extra time within each movement so that the tasks are successfully completed by those who need more time. That additional time also yields additional reflection on the theme, on the moments in the script, and on the lives participants are living in their recovery. Further studies should consider increasing the number of participants and the number of productions for persons with aphasia. A comprehensive look at the difference between aphasia treatment as usual and aphasia treatment in tandem with CoATT would be beneficial.

We imagine a community in which CPs work closely with speech-language pathologists and their respective centers, and alongside caregivers of persons with aphasia. We can see a space in which CoATT fills the gap in the psychosocial needs regarding connection and identity, bringing innovation and fun to rote aspects of language re-learning.

Reference List

Boal, A. (1974). 1979. Theater of the oppressed.

Cahana-Amitay, D., & Albert, M. L. (2015). *Redefining recovery from aphasia*. Oxford University Press.

Code, C. (2001). Multifactorial processes in recovery from aphasia: Developing the foundations for a multileveled framework. *Brain and Language, 77*(1): 25–44. 10. 1006/brln.2000.2420

Code, C., & Herrmann, M. (2003). The relevance of emotional and psychosocial factors in aphasia to rehabilitation. *Neuropsychological Rehabilitation, 13*(1–2): 109–132. 10.1080/09602010244000291

Coelho, P. (2007, December 10). The Lesson of the Butterfly. Paulo Coelho: Stories and reflections. https://paulocoelhoblog.com/2007/12/10/the-lesson-of-the-butterfly/

Cruice, M., Worrall, L., Hickson, L., & Murison, R. (2003). Finding a focus for quality of life with aphasia: Social and emotional health, and psychological well-being. *Aphasiology, 17*(4): 333–353. 10.1080/02687030244000707

Datta, H., Wood, L. L., Alimonti, S. H., Pugliese, D., Butkiewicz, H., Jannello, F., Rissland, B., & Tully, K. (in press). Audience and caregiver responses to witnessing persons with aphasia participate in coactive therapeutic theater: A mixed methods study. *International Journal of Language and Communication Disorders*.

Dalemans, R. J., de Witte, L., Wade, D., & van den Heuvel, W. (2010). Social participation through the eyes of people with aphasia. *International Journal of Language & Communication Disorders, 45*(5): 537–550. Palgrave Macmillan. 10.3109/1368282 0903223633

Meisner, S., & Longwell, D. (1987). *Sanford meisner on acting*. Vintage Books.

National Aphasia Alliance. 2016. *Home Page*. https://www.aphasia.org

Ross, K., & Wertz, R. (2003). Quality of life with and without aphasia. *Aphasiology*, *17*(4): 355–364. 10.1080/02687030244000716

Simmons-Mackie, N., & Damico, J. S. (2011). Counseling and aphasia treatment: Missed opportunities. *Topics in Language Disorders*, *31*(4): 336–351. 10.1097/TLD.0b013e318234ea9f

Wood, L. L., Bryant, D., Scirocco, K., Datta, H., Alimonti, S., & Mowers, D. (2020). Aphasia Park: A pilot study using the co-active therapeutic theater model with clients in aphasia recovery. *The Arts in Psychotherapy*, *67*: Article 101611. 10.1016/j.aip.2019.101611

Chapter 7

Learning from the Scripts

Previous chapters presented a CoATT script with notations that describe the processes of rehearsal and performance alongside the script of the play. The dynamic of play development was revealed alongside a discussion of the ways in which recovery is strengthened for participants. The explication draws on the specific relationships between the metaphoric material of the play and the material of participants in treatment. This also approximates the view of the CoATT practitioner. The manualized exercises create a structure, the participants provide material, and the process of playmaking unfolds in real-time with the group. The experience of opening night, however, is different for an audience member who has simply come to see a play.

It is one of the most distinct features of CoATT that a public performance will include audience members who have a tangential relationship to the cast, or to the subject matter of their recovery. This means that the metaphors contained in the play must be independently compelling and sound, the production values clear and appropriate, and the theme of the performance meaningful and valuable. Staging such an event requires that a CP thinks deeply about the play itself and allows the audience to do so as well.

The notion of studying plays could suggest interpretation of the material for dramatic presentation, or alternative meaning and artistic value. The CoATT plays are not intended to exist as great plays, *per se*, but as the outcome of the group process. These plays will have more power in the community event of public performance and memorialize the achievement of constructing a drama that holds meaning for the group and the audience.

We have included two additional CoATT scripts with discussion questions, both of which were built using the manualized model. This chapter, and the questions following each script, explore the relationship between the execution of a script and the reception of the audience. The exercise may be useful in understanding the recovery of these unique groups.

One play came from a group of individuals who were diagnosed with schizophrenia and who had some challenges with line memorization, movement, and sustained concentration. The play also took place online, due to the COVID-19 pandemic. The other play came from adult participants who

DOI: 10.4324/9781003161608-8

had strong communication and movement skills but were also diagnosed with a substance use disorder. In both cases, the audience simply sat down to encounter a play and make sense of it for themselves. A clear reading of these plays may help simulate that experience. Reading the play aloud with a group will enhance understanding and call upon embodied experiences.

Play 1: Lost and Found

Introduction and Participants

UMass Mind is a community outreach program at the University of Massachusetts Medical School in Worcester, focusing on psychotic disorders. In 2020, working in partnership with the authors, the program received a grant from the U.S.-based National Endowment for the Arts. The grant proposal matched the CoATT model with the institution's population of individuals with "serious and persistent mental illness." The study was intended to be the first Randomized Control Trial (RCT) with the model, and we had planned to produce five plays over the course of three years, while also running a treatment-as-usual (TAU) group. As we were preparing to start our first production, COVID-19 hit the United States and effectively shut down any hope of live theatre.

In discussing this dilemma, we wondered if the CoATT model would work online. Was it wise to try applying CoATT to a new population in a new setting with a new treatment facility as sponsor? Because we had some experience working with schizophrenia in other contexts, we agreed to pursue this new type of production. Everyone involved with the grant remained convinced this online experience would be a one-off project. Likely, by the time the second production would start, we would be back in person and in theatres. COVID-19 would run its course and live performance would allow us to return to the original conception of the model.

Working with drama therapy interns Emily and Francesca, we adapted the exercises for Zoom. Surprisingly, the exercises worked fairly well in the online format. Our major takeaway was to ensure session times remained manageable to accommodate "Zoom fatigue," which was compounded by some members' medication side effects.

The cast was made up of seven individuals – two women and five men – with schizophrenia diagnoses. The group deemed that their definition of active recovery included being in relationships through offering support and being supported by others. The group was very clear that hearing or seeing things that other people did not hear or see was, at times, a part of their lives. They agreed that coaching and supporting each other through those moments, without sharing details about what they were seeing or hearing, was very important. Early on, the group answered the CoATT Question with a powerful concept: Hope is necessary to sustaining mental wellness.

Sub-themes involved the concepts of "chosen family" and "non-judgment," with an emphasis on destigmatizing mental illness. One member of the group didn't resonate with this concept of recovery and decided to leave. This pattern is not unfamiliar in a CoATT process. However, group members usually stay and work through challenges as part of the model. We offer the play itself as a way to hold the paradoxes and multiple truths present for cast members. In this case, the individual who left early was unwilling to come back and consider this possibility. For him, protecting his recovery during the pandemic meant not participating in the group.

The remaining group worked in harmony. They supported each other during challenging moments, validated one another's voices, and were energized by coming back to the CoATT Question. The group enjoyed working in a fantasy realm. But to stabilize individuals who may struggle to differentiate fantasy and reality, each session included additional clarity in moments of entering and exiting a play space (Pendzik, 2016). Already skilled at reality testing for themselves and others, the group incorporated this step with ease. This finding surprised both the medical students and CPs. The literature on schizophrenia often indicates that reality testing is the preferred approach for treatment and that playing with fantasy and reality is counter-indicated (Kopelovich & Turkington, 2021). With the addition of clear entry and exit into dramatic reality and extended de-roling, the participants were able to begin to play with the idea of fantasy and found a lot of enjoyment from it. Their fantasy realm allowed kings, queens, and royal family to emerge as characters.

The biggest challenges for most group members were technical issues. We were lucky to have some first-year medical students supporting the project, and they were able to help troubleshoot. Ensuring people had access to technology beyond their phones was critical to successful work in a virtual setting.

Given the level of focus and Zoom fatigue, the team delivered the absolute bare minimum of exercises to maintain fidelity to the Intensive movement. The CoATT team decided to discontinue the homework assignments from that point, however, as they placed a heavy demand on the group during an already challenging time. Notably, homework assignments in the Rehearsal movement of the model are operationalized as reflections on the process. While this reflection time may have been stabilizing or beneficial in other ways, the group and CoATT team agreed that dropping them would not affect the development of the play itself. As with any therapeutic undertaking, the participants set the pace of work and therapists worked to adapt the demand to the group's needs and abilities.

In most CoATT productions the cast is disappointed with the script when first presented with it. The big emotional release mobilizes the group to edit and take ownership of the work. With this cast, the group had crystalized their theme and worked hard to develop their roles during the Intensive. The writing of the script happened relatively quickly, and the group felt pleased overall, with only minor edits to some language to help it sound more natural. One notable dynamic was the change of assigned character names to new names that spoke more to each actor. The play was set in a Zoom room, which made acting choices accessible and removed set and prop requirements. Complex entrances and exits were eliminated. In rehearsal, participants learned to improvise when tech issues or microphone issues arose. As expected, these same technical challenges arose during the performance. For example, the Zoom Room Operator, played by one of the CP interns, could jokingly say, "Queen Regina, please unmute!" When this occurred, the participants added dramatic slapstick reactions, acting as if the moment had been rehearsed. This blurring of the line between reality and dramatic reality was particularly poignant for the medical students and drama therapy CP interns. The participants demonstrated the ways in which the dominant narrative "truths" that we often force on individuals with schizophrenia can both be true and not true.

Two important discoveries emerged during the rehearsal movement. First, it became important to have the participants' actual names next to their character names in the script. This allowed them to track the script more easily, as well as enroll and de-role. This technique emphasizes the paradox of "me" and "not me" when stepping into a role (Landy, 1994). It also serves to keep participants grounded in the action of the dramatic reality. Second, given some of the participants' medication side effects and life circumstances, this cast struggled to memorize the script. Working on Zoom became a gift because participants could get the gist of their lines, but look down to their script, if need be, while still appearing to have memorized their lines to those watching on screen. The group delighted in ways to hide their scripts – such as hanging them on the wall or hiding them in a prop book –that made sense in the context of the play.

The collusion between the participants, who are actors in the play, and the CoATT team, who are directors or presenters in this moment, is meant to mimic a traditional theatrical presentation where actors know their lines and say them as if speaking the spontaneous thoughts of their characters. It is important to note that the intention of the group was not to mask their schizophrenia but rather to make their performance as accessible as possible for an audience expecting a traditional play. The essence of reconnection with one's community is sharing a reality. In this case, the audience and performers have agreed to the dramatic reality that these are characters speaking spontaneously rather than reading a script. They've found a simple but profound way to connect.

The online play performed with success in the Zoom theatre world. The significant reach of Zoom allowed participants to have many friends, family, treatment team members, and unknown "users," join as a public audience. Many people living with chronic mental health issues struggle to participate in large community gatherings, but technology creates access. Access builds equity for all community members. Zoom as a connective technology was "thrilling" for the extended community. Participants led the co-active audience element using the chat feature. Zoom technology allows the team to record and save both the performance and audience chat. This important artifact became a prompt during the Launch movement.

The results of the study are to be co-authored with the University Medical and research teams. One emerging qualitative finding was that group members felt working on Zoom was a benefit; the participants expressed hope that when the pandemic did resolve, this delivery format could be adapted as an ongoing option. Like other CoATT groups, participants cited the connections they made with peers and credited the unique approach to treatment offered by the CoATT model.

Script

LOST AND FOUND
_____

Created by a group working on mental wellness recovery in

2020

CAST OF CHARACTERS

ZOOM ROOM OPERATOR................................Franny
QUEEN REGINA.......................................Kelly
KERMIT...Wayne
MR. BOB..Has
AUSTIN..Denver
REBEL...Mirabelle
SISSY..Meredith
BROTHER MIKE....................................Mitchel

AT RISE: "Lights Up." The audience sees one
                                person on the Zoom screen. Her name
                                reads "Zoom Room Operator." She is
                                wearing a headset, dressed in a
                                white button up shirt and wears a
                                pair of black rimmed glasses. She is
                                professional and eager. Suddenly,
                                we hear an *ding-dong* sound,
                                alerting us a person is joining. A
                                new zoom box appears, joining the
                                Zoom Room Operator, the name reads
                                "Queen Regina." She wears a beau-
                                tiful crown and is dressed regally.
                                She is optimistic and reliable.

QUEEN REGINA
I am Her Majesty, Queen Regina! I am so pleased to meet you
all …
                (She looks around and realizes that nobody is here
                expect for the ZOOM ROOM OPERATOR.)

Where is everyone? I got an invitation that said I was going
to be honored today for being a compassionate ruler.
                (Sound cue of Zoom Alert.)

OPERATOR
Standby please, another guest is entering.

                    QUEEN REGINA
Harumph. Well, can I at least have a biscuit while I wait?

> (She takes out a biscuit from her purse and
> eats it.)

                    KERMIT
Hello! I'm Kermit, the great wise leader. I'm here in the
zoom room to lead a presentation today for you all on the keys
to finding wisdom and happiness.

> (He looks around confused and says:)

                    KERMIT
Where are all the people?

                    QUEEN REGINA
Wait one minute, what did you get an invite for?

                    KERMIT
I got an invite to come give a talk on the keys to finding
wisdom and happiness to help people.

> (They look to the ZOOM ROOM OPERATOR and both say:)

                    QUEEN REGINA AND KERMIT
Operator, what's going on here?

> (Sound cue of Zoom Alert.)

                    OPERATOR
Standby please, another guest is entering.

> (Enter BROTHER MIKE)

                    BROTHER
Hey my fellow Worcester people!

                    QUEEN REGINA
I'm not from Worcester, I'm the Queen of Croatia!

                    KERMIT
I'm not from Worcester, I'm a great wise leader.

> (They look to the ZOOM ROOM OPERATOR and both say:)

                    QUEEN REGINA AND KERMIT AND BROTHER
What's going on here?

                    OPERATOR
Standby please, another guest is entering.

> (Sound cue of Zoom Alert.)

> (Enter BOB.)

                         BOB
Hey everyone, I'm so glad that you're here to receive the
peace and love … .

              (They cut him off.)

                    QUEEN REGINA AND KERMIT AND BROTHER
WE'RE NOT!

                    QUEEN REGINA
I mean, we are … but there has been a mix-up. Zoom Operator,
can you please tell us what's going on?

              (Sound cue of Zoom Alert.)

              (The group throws their hands up in frustration.)

                    OPERATOR
Standby please, another guest is entering.

              (Enter KING AUSTIN.)

                    KING AUSTIN
It is I, your royal highness, King Austin.

                    QUEEN REGINA
Let me guess, you got an invitation saying you were going to
be honored for being a compassionate leader?

                    KING AUSTIN
Why, that's exactly right … is this not the ceremony honoring me?

                    EVERYONE
NO!

              (Sound cue of Zoom Alert.)

              (The group puts their heads in their hands.)

                    OPERATOR
Standby please, another guest is entering.

              (Enter REBEL, she sees everyone looks frus-
              trated.)

                    REBEL
Well, aren't you all a friendly group …

              (Sound cue of Zoom Alert.)

                    OPERATOR
Standby please, another guest is entering.

                    QUEEN REGINA
This is ridiculous.

          (SISSY enters.)
                    SISSY
Hey y'all, what's up?

                    QUEEN REGINA
I'll tell you what's up. Someone has sent a Zoom invitation
to each of us, requesting our presence for various different
reasons. This must be some kind of a joke?

                    SISSY
It couldn't be a joke!

                    OPERATOR
I can assure you this is no joke! I am a very experienced …
Zoom operator … and I can assure I have been paid a great deal
of money to ensure this goes well!

                    QUEEN REGINA
I hope so! I was very busy running my kingdom, which I've
spent many years preparing for since my adoption into the
royal family when I was four. I've been studying for years to
finally take over the royal duties and always have had a
compassionate approach. Not ruling with an iron fist, but a
compassionate heart. So, while I'm sure you all are lovely,
I do really need to get back to my people.

                    KING AUSTIN
Wait a minute, you were adopted? I was also adopted by a royal
family when I was 4.

                    REBEL
Wait a minute, this is very strange. I'm also royalty but
I've been all alone on my island, the Island of Monroe, which
I've been the princess of since I was four.

                    KERMIT
Never fear … I'm a wise leader so rest assured, I will figure
this out!

                    BOB
Hey man, I'm also a wise leader.

                    KERMIT
Well, I've actually been a wise leader to royalty …

                              BOB
Hey man, no need to brag. I also have been a wise advisor to
royalty.

          (The QUEEN turns to the ZOOM ROOM OPERATOR.)

                         QUEEN REGINA
Zoom Operator, what is going on here?!

                            OPERATOR
Well, it seems that everyone has received an invitation
inviting them to a different event. And now, we have a room
full of royalty, three of which were adopted at the age of
four and two former royal advisors.

               (The QUEEN looks to SISSY.)

                         QUEEN REGINA
And you? Who are you? Are you also the ruler of a kingdom?

                             SISSY
Well, I'm sort of from a kingdom. The animal kingdom. What I
mean is I work at the zoo. In Hawaii. I work with the big cats.

                              BOB
                    (Strokes his beard)

Curiouser and curiouser.

                            KERMIT
Hey … I was gonna say that.

                         QUEEN REGINA
And you, Mike? Who are you? Also from a kingdom I suppose?

                            BROTHER
I'm not from any Kingdom. I'm from Worcester. But I'm
picking up on a pattern here. So, the three of you royals were
all were adopted at the age of four. Don't you think that is
an odd coincidence and now you are all here? What happened
before that?

                            KERMIT
I was just about to ask just that!

                         QUEEN REGINA
Well of course, 35 years ago there was a great war. My parents
were forced to give me up for adoption. I don't remember much
about it, I was so little.

                         KING AUSTIN
Me too!

                         REBEL
Me three!

                         BOB
            (Strokes his beard)
Curiouser and curiouser.

                         KERMIT
I was gonna say that!

                         BROTHER
Well … I'm no advisor to the king but seems to me that we're
onto something.

                         BOB
Well, in times like these, I always call upon a message of
hope to get through times of confusion: Hope is always
there. There is always hope for you. When the time is right,
love is the way. Love is the way, when the time is right.

                         KERMIT
I was gonna say that!

                         BOB
Now wait just a minute. How were you possibly going to say
that? Those are the sacred words of King Zaban. May he rest in
peace.

                         KERMIT
King Zaban? Don't you mean Queen Zaban? Who, might I add, I
personally worked for as the royal advisor. I helped advise
her on building beautiful places for people to find meaning
in their lives.

                         BOB
Wait! You worked for Queen Zaban?

                         KERMIT
Yes – that's what I just said!

            (A beat.)

                         KERMIT
Wait a moment – you worked for King Zaban?!

                    ALL (EXCEPT KERMIT AND BOB)
Curiouser and curiouser.

KERMIT

Hey! I was gonna say …

BROTHER

We know, we know, you were gonna say that. So, you both worked for the same royal couple?

BOB

Not only did I work for King Zaban as his wise advisor, but he was also my brother.

BROTHER

Let me guess, Kermit … you were also …

ALL

The queen's brother!

SISSY

I knew you all could figure it out.

> (She looks at QUEEN REGINA, PRINCESS REBEL and KING AUSTIN.)

QUEEN REGINA

Sissy?

KING AUSTIN

Sissy!

REBEL

It's our Sister- Sissy!

QUEEN REGINA

I remember … I had an older sister … WE had an older sister. Could it be true?

SISSY

Yes … and you three, the triplets- Regina, Austin, Rebel. I've missed you so much. And I've kept you here, close to my heart. The only picture of us all I keep here in this locket … my family.

> (She opens the locket and holds up a photo.)

QUEEN REGINA

But how?

SISSY

In my spare time between working at the zoo and enjoying the beaches of Hawaii, I started studying genealogy. I took a class with Dr. Witnesson, who is an expert in long-lost royal family relationships.

QUEEN REGINA

Who on earth is Dr. Whitson?

(The ZOOM ROOM OPERATOR removes her glasses.)

(The group gasps.)

OPERATOR

on Instagram, Twitter and Facebook. Thank you.

I'm actually not a Zoom operator at all. It is I, Dr. Cecelia Witnesson, Professor of Genealogy and author of renowned book "Finding Your Lost Royal Family: Messengers of Hope Are Born and Made," available on Amazon or at your local bookstore. Check me out at www.Dr.Whitnessonreveals

(The ZOOM ROOM OPERATOR bows.)

QUEEN REGINA

My goodness. You did all this for your book? For fame and accolades …

OPERATOR

No, no – you've got it all wrong! When Sissy called me from Hawaii and told me this story – I knew there was something so important here! I said "Yes! I will take this case on – these people are going to change the word!" Such a powerful family separated at birth by a terrible war scattered to the winds! But you can never just tell people the obvious – they have to figure it out for themselves! So – I began to search to put the mystery together. Allow me to share.

(She screen shares the family tree.)

OPERATOR

You see, first I discovered that Queen Regina had ended up in Croatia where she was celebrated to be a compassionate leader, so that was an easy invite to make up. And it should come as no surprise that her brother, King Austin, was ALSO a compassionate leader and that I could send him an invite stating the same thing. Now, tracking down Princess Rebel was a little easier, but as I was flying around searching for her, she was easy to spot in her pink and black spandex outfit on her own island. Then it was easy to tell our two wise advisor Uncles that they were giving a special talk on helping people, and then Sissy just had to stay quiet when everyone entered and then VOILA! I knew it would merely be a matter of time before you all would put it together!!!

> (She takes a bow and the group claps in astonishment.)

BOB
Wait a minute! If the Zoom operator is actually Professor Witnesson, then who are you?

> (Points to BROTHER MIKE.)

KERMIT
I was gonna say that!

BROTHER
I don't know how I got here. I'm just a guy from Worcester. I don't have a great story with my family. I was the black sheep of the family. My family wasn't kind or loving or compassionate to me. And for a while I got really lost. I didn't know what was real and what wasn't. But I got myself out. I did it by having a good attitude, good beliefs, and asking for help. Now I know what's real and what's not. Although I don't have a family. I have a group that I'm a part of, which is what I thought this invitation was for tonight. But guess I somehow just got the wrong link.

REBEL
I've always wanted a brother who was a black sheep to join me, the rebel princess.

KING AUSTIN
I didn't even know I had siblings until today, but having a brother to help me out with all this sister energy is probably going to come in handy.

QUEEN REGINA
Even if you're not my brother by blood, you could be a brother in my heart. A heart brother.

SISSY
Would you join our family, Brother Mike?

BROTHER
I'd like that. Plus, I'd love to have you all come to Worcester.

SISSY

My dream has come true. Not about Worcester … I mean … Here we are together, our first family reunion. It makes me so happy; I just want to dance!

(Cue music. "Everybody Dance Now" plays. The group dances.)

(The music stops. Everybody is laughing and feeling good.)

OPERATOR

I'm sorry to say but your time limit on zoom is running out.

(The group is disappointed.)

QUEEN REGINA

Oh no. I hate goodbyes.

SISSY

The good news is even though we are out of time today, we have each other now. We have our amazing, strong royal family.

QUEEN REGINA

That's true, Sissy. And you know, being with you all, I have a newfound sense of hope. I feel more optimistic than ever.

BOB

Ah, well … Hope is always there. There is always hope for you KERMIT … ...When the time is right, love is the way.

BROTHER

Love is the way, when the time is right.

SISSY

A message of hope.

KING AUSTIN

It's exactly what I needed to hear today and I'm going to take it back to my people.

QUEEN REGINA

Me too.

REBEL

Me three. But I better write that down so I don't forget.

(They all write it down on paper. They all hold it up to the camera and say it together.)

REBEL, AUSTIN, REGINA

Hope is always there. There is always hope for you. When the time is right, love is the way. Love is the way, when the time is right.

(Cut to black. All actors turn off their Zoom video, leaving the ZOOM ROOM OPERATOR alone. She brings back each actor to the screen one by one. Each person says, "My name is _____ and today I played the role of _____.)

(Final bows.)

(Group facilitates co-active element with audience.)

(END OF PLAY)

Discussion Questions

1 CoATT participants must identify themselves as "in active recovery." What evidence of active recovery is found in the script? Are there instructions for living that support an active recovery?

2 The Zoom Room Operator plays a major role. How does this character function to keep the action of the play moving forward? How does this character figure in the emotional journey of each character? How does the role of the operator parallel the role of a therapist?

3 Family is a central metaphor in the play. How does family figure into a healthy recovery? What wisdom does the play contain for family members of people in recovery?

4 This play was created during the COVID-19 crisis. What elements of the production represent successful adaptation to quarantine? What impact does that have on relationships between the characters? How might this impact the relationship between actors? What benefits might this population derive from adapting the play to Zoom? What benefits may be lost?

5 Can you think of a model for this script? What sources in popular culture might have influenced the script? What other stories or forms does this play remind you of?

6 What do the characters have in common? How does it parallel what a group in recovery might have in common?

7 Croatia is an actual country but does not have a monarchy. In what way is this a challenge to reality testing for a group living with chronic, persistent mental illness? What benefit might be gained by correcting this? Why might a group leave this unaddressed?

Play 2: Paths of the Prism

Introduction and Participants

CoATT productions operate with the principle that participants hold, and share, a working definition of "active recovery." In a group that shares a long treatment process, language describing the concept might easily gel, including a set of daily activities that support active recovery. When the recovery is defined by the medical model it might include behavior guidelines such as abstaining from self-harm for chronic and persistent mental illness or using an expanded number of words in spontaneous conversation for those with aphasia. The shared understanding of active recovery is fertile ground for the imagination when a group is in the generation movement of CoATT process, allowing all participants to celebrate a certain type of moment or collectively push back against a familiar challenge. But when a group comes together with strongly divergent conceptions of active recovery, the Generation tasks can take on a stormy quality or leave the CoATT practitioners with widely disparate scenes, characters, and monologues from which to make the play. This was the case with the substance use disorder pilot group that created the play, *Paths of the Prism.*

The pilot program was sponsored by two recovery treatment centers in a distant suburb of New York City. Participants were recruited from members of a day treatment program operating as part of a Catholic health services hospital and from a "sober house" step-down program for people in recovery from drug and alcohol addiction. Drama therapy interns under Laura's supervision led CoATT-inspired group drama therapy sessions weekly on-site at the day treatment center for four months prior to the formal CoATT production. Participants made a 14-week commitment to attend all groups. Interested group members volunteered to participate in the public performance held off-site at the hospital's conference facility. That group had six men and three women ranging in age from late twenties to early fifties. The racial make-up of the group included two Black individuals, one Latinx person, and six participants identifying as White. With the exception of one Black woman (who self-reported that they questioned their gender identity), the participants were local to the suburban setting. All participants had been to "rehab" at least once, and most had a strong personal definition of their "active recovery."

The six men in the group were living in the sober house with varying levels of sobriety time, meaning that they tested negative for substances daily as a condition of their residence. Other conditions for staying in the house included attending a daily Alcoholics Anonymous (AA) meeting and a daily house meeting. One of the women in the group lived in a similar sober house for women; the others lived in the community. The daily abstention from substance use was a condition of the day treatment program as well. All participants had a shared understanding of "active recovery" that included physical sobriety and abstention from the use of all illicit substances.

But that was where the shared conception ended. Group members had divergent opinions and understanding of the AA program.

According to their literature, AA as an organization has no opinion on outside matters, including other treatment modalities or programs, and it defines itself as "a fellowship of people who share their experience, strength and hope with each other that they may solve their common problem and help others to recover from alcoholism" (Alcoholics Anonymous, 2021). It offers "twelve steps that are suggested as a program of recovery" (Alcoholics Anonymous, 2002, p. 52) without insistence on any member taking those steps. These steps include reference to a "higher power" or "power greater than oneself" to support recovery, and stress building a relationship with "God, as we understood him" (p. 52). The book, *Alcoholics Anonymous*, goes further, in a chapter titled "We Agnostics," to emphasize that there is no requirement to believe in God or follow the dogma of the program. One tradition that underpins all AA groups is that "the only requirement for membership is a desire to stop drinking" (p. 562).

The AA program is carried into the community by untrained, unlicensed, non-professional group members, so even direct statements from the literature may take on the flavor of the group in question. For many people, the language is charged by negative experiences with organized religion, temperance programs, or previous treatment, and those elements may leak into the AA group process. It is uncommon to find a perfectly harmonious and completely aligned meeting of AA. Compulsory attendance does little to build a sense of acceptance of the program.

This was the case with our participants. For those members living in the halfway house, discussions about the AA program and principles spilled into the day treatment setting. Arguments that began in the morning meeting at the house continued through drama-therapy group and reappeared in the evening CoATT sessions. The central tension in the argument centered on dogma: Is sobriety contingent on doing and saying what the AA program tells you? A secondary argument focused on 'belief in a higher power" but lacked the same charged emotional force. Instead, the group adopted a "choose your own higher power" stance, demonstrating tolerance for Jewish traditions, Catholic teachings, evangelical experience, and agnosticism.

Writing assignments brought this division into stark relief as CP1 collected artifacts from the group. Some participants submitted long monologues culled directly from AA literature when asked to write "as your Recovery." Others cribbed from secular sources, taking passages of poetry and inspirational literature they came across in treatment. Scenes often devolved into barely veiled one-on-one arguments in which one character had to lose in order for another to win. These argument scenes could be read as substitutions for "there's only one way to get sober." Authoritarian characters appeared, announcing "my way or the highway."

The most senior member of the sober house was also the most vocal about AA as the sole path to recovery. In scene work, he spouted dogma, and in interpersonal interactions adopted a fierce pro-AA position. Two of the other men sparred with him in jest, engaging him with humor about his rigidity while acknowledging his leadership in the group. The banter sounded like an old-fashioned comedic routine that lent itself naturally to scene improvisations. From this dynamic, a leading character emerged: the Great Horn, a God with all the answers.

Most members of the group had a concrete understanding of what their lives in recovery might look like. This is to say that they could imagine circumstances they hoped would surround them but could not quite articulate the scaffolding they might need to build those realities on a bedrock of sobriety. When prompted to speak "as" their own Recovery, the tendency in the group was to give descriptions of current problems solved or personal situations improved. One woman imagined herself as a "better mother," perhaps reunited with her estranged children through her grandchildren. Another member imagined himself with a successful acting career. One senior member was actively working on joining a union and landing steady work. Another concrete goal was stable and independent housing, which had as much to do with "escaping the halfway house" as demonstrating achievement.

These individual projections played out during the Intensive weekend rehearsals. By joining in to play a variety of roles as we worked through the multiple storylines, members made a strong demonstration of support for each other's recovery. In order to create some distance from the psychodramatic content in these scenes, the cast experimented with fictionalizing names, creating characters, and looking for connections between stories.

Uniting the individual stories around a theme proved problematic. There was great material between the Great Horn and his challengers. The scenes played at a brisk pace, had funny jokes with punchlines, and commented directly on recovery techniques. Still, the Great Horn – both the character *and* the actor tapped to play him – remained essentially non-dramatic and unable to change his dogmatic views. Two stories linked on themes of family reunification; two other stories were about the "pursuit of my true self." But no single story or theme satisfied even a majority of group members.

Repeated attempts were made to come back to the CoATT Question: "What is a theme of recovery you want to create a play about in service of strengthening your recovery and sharing with an audience?" Many truths were generated, but the group was unable even to rank them with a vote. Finally, the group member who was working on a story of "finding himself as an artist" and adamantly rejected AA dogma offered a summation: "There is no one way to achieve recovery, it's different for all of us." This became the theme of the play, reflected in the title *Paths of the Prism*.

In the role of CP2, Dave spent time on the material that had been gathered during the Generation phase to prepare for the Intensive weekend. Successful CoATT practitioners find inspiration in their study of dramatic literature and pop culture, often borrowing plots or storylines for use in drama therapy productions. Here, Shakespeare provided models that wove together multiple narratives and knitted up the actions between gods and mankind.

- Two Artist characters were looking to find themselves out in the world of recovery, calling to mind Viola and Sebastian searching for each other in Shakespeare's Twelfth Night.
- The mother figure who emerged in scene work was seeking the restoration of her family, hoping for a kind of passive reconnection to the children she felt she had "lost' in her addiction. The Abbess in *Comedy of Errors* is reunited with her children, proving their connection with a cherished artifact after the family is thrown back together in Syracuse.
- Shakespeare's comedies often call upon the gods to direct a wedding, suggesting the Great Horn might direct the reunion in *Paths of the Prism*, but that trope would underline the message that dogma contains the correct formula for happy resolutions. Besides, the fun of the Great Horn sequences arose from the conflict and argument surrounding him. In *The Tempest,* Prospero influences the action on the island and seas around him while balancing the elemental forces of Ariel and Caliban.

Another storyline from the group focused on the career and success of the youngest participant, a man in his early twenties intent on becoming a performer. While he was comfortable speculating about what kind of musician or actor he could become, he was more interested in re-telling the stories of how his addiction had undermined his potential than imagining a path forward. In terms of his treatment, he was working in groups and therapy on Mourning and Remembrance, playing and replaying his past mistakes. During discussion in the Intensive weekend the participants named this dynamic "remaining trapped in the past." For the two group members who declined the dogma of AA in favor of the Artist role, resolution of this tension was expected in a moment of "sober inspiration" that would finally move an Artist to "find themselves" and "make the world better through art."

The world of *Paths of the Prism* began to come into focus with problems in a "heavenly realm" between the Great Horn and his minions, and earthly struggles below as siblings and parents yearned to find themselves, find each other, and make something of their lives. Yet the link between worlds remained elusive, and the debate amongst the gods remained stagnant. Replaying the autobiographically inspired scenes of failure had the group thinking of flashbacks and alternate realities in which the course of fate can be altered. It's a common trope in American films. The group wondered, "If the Great Horn is a god, why can't he go in or go back and change things?" Refusing to allow the dogma-derived deity to demonstrate his powers for good prioritized the belief of those participants who rejected dogma altogether. Linking the powers of the gods to the hearts and destinies of folks on earth became a stumbling block.

The solution was suggested by a beloved American film, *It's a Wonderful Life (Capra, 1946),* in which an imperfect angel called Clarence must earn his wings by saving the life and spirit of a small-town banker called George Bailey. The useful premise for *Paths of the Prism* is that the angel has a motivation for intervening in the affairs of men; he isn't an eternally fixed and perfect being, rather, he's trying to better himself. This created a dramatic link and a reason for the two realms in the world of the play to interact. Additionally, it underlined a dynamic of 12-step recovery programs. The messengers may be imperfect, but you may find value in the experience of working with others. If so, all are welcome to pursue their recovery.

Ultimately, the presentation of the script devised in the Intensive weekend took a much different form than expected. Early in the process, a female member dropped out of the group by relapsing and leaving treatment. The script was developed to incorporate her early contributions, with processing in group time devoted to the idea that relapse does not negate a person or her sober work and contributions. The group celebrated her contributions and remembered her as an important part of each of their journeys, and a CP intern took on the role, holding her spirit and presence.

During rehearsal, more cast changes took place. The participant who wrote and performed the Great Horn decided not to continue with the play. His stated reasons included that the script trivialized AA literature, offered counter-productive messages about recovery, and created a bad dynamic in the sober house with only some members receiving the perks of being a cast member. No amount of counseling, rewriting, or negotiation could ensure his return. With time short and a dwindling cast, CP2 (Dave) stepped in to play the Great Horn. In performance, this placed the therapist in a truly co-active mode as rehearsals, rewrites, and real-time coaching on sobriety condensed into an even more intimate connection. CP1(Laura) kept the focus of rehearsals on recovery with the question: "How is this experience of rehearsing the play and losing an actor like recovery?"

Participants had an answer at the ready: "While you are doing your recovery in the course of your life, people will come and go, even important ones, but your sobriety is your own. You must find a way to keep going and maintain your recovery." Then a third actor dropped out. The individual playing one of the Artist protagonists went missing from the halfway house. Cast members were certain that they had left to use drugs and alcohol; the facility attempted to trace their whereabouts but could not. The group experienced this loss perhaps more deeply than when the Great Horn dropped out. He was still a leader at the halfway house and demonstrating his sobriety. This latest lost cast member may have been literally lost to addiction or foul play on the streets. The group paused rehearsals to acknowledge the real-life stakes of recovery. The treatment facility and CoATT team made what efforts they could to locate the individual and ensure their safety. When they were found, they were invited to attend the performance, but declined to attend.

When the fourth cast member, the man playing an Artist and Angel, went missing from the halfway house, the group went into crisis mode. The facilities (both halfway house and hospital day treatment program) expressed concern that the CoATT production was to blame. This participant, however, made it clear that it was interpersonal conflict at the halfway house, a sense of being alone, and frustration with the dogma of treatment that caused him to leave. He signed out and went home to his community; he did not promise to return, neither did he promise to complete the production. He did, however, take phone calls from CP1. He stated that the play gave him meaning and a purpose, and he wanted to fulfill his role as an artist.

The team running CoATT assured him that the role was his, and he needed only to return to group physically sober to continue rehearsals. The facilities had a more difficult time accepting that a patient (in the medical model, of course, "patient" terminology dominates over "participant") might come and go against advice. Institutions often threaten an adverse consequence for disobeying rules and recommendations. The participant assured everyone that he was not drinking or using drugs. Medical staff admitted to doubting him. Participants worried that any addict or alcoholic would have a hard time staying sober or telling the truth about relapse. The CoATT team hoped for the best while scrambling to cover the role. At this point, the female dramatherapy intern was covering a role and CP2 was covering the Great Horn. There was no one left to cover the role without a massive overhaul of the script. Production was three weeks away.

Technical rehearsals and run-throughs began three days prior to the public performance. The errant Angel arrived for rehearsal, having cleared his physical and drug tests, and with the reluctant blessing of his day program. He would not be re-admitted to the halfway house, nor did he wish to be. The group welcomed him back and he stepped directly into rehearsal. The CoATT team offered the group a chance to process his return; the unanimous decision was to welcome him back to work with little fanfare. When asked how this situation might mirror their future recovery, the group pointed to the message of the play: Everyone has to do recovery their own way.

This participant, vocal and committed to his belief that he could find and maintain his own recovery without dogma, created for himself a real-life experience of his character's belief. While he was away from the group, he continued to write poetry that he hoped might become lyrics or find publication. He identified *Paths of the Prism* as a moment of inspiration and, because he remained sober, he knew he could benefit from returning to the production to express himself as an artist.

In production, *Paths of the Prism* took on elements of classical psychodrama as well as Boal's Theatre of the Oppressed. With drama therapists stepping into roles, several participants played scenes with trained Auxiliaries. The Mother got to embrace a CP intern, now portraying her lost daughter; the young man recreating his failures got to play through these memories opposite CP2, rehearsing new strategies for the future. In the final moments of the play, as the Great Horn, CP2 asked the participant, as Joseph, an angel of inspiration to artists, "What do you see ahead?" Both character and actor spoke his answer, written by the group and rehearsed for many weeks, with new resonance, "It's the path. I see the path."

The script for *Paths of the Prism* does not capture the healing of the process, nor does it contain great playwriting, *per se*. But it does capture the manifold and tumultuous journey toward recovery from substance use disorder as described by a variety of individuals bound together with the shared experience of only a few weeks at the very beginning of their sober lives. In that way the script is a clear mirror of most treatment groups; each individual struggles to understand their own experience and to make their way forward using new behaviors. The process of rehearsing and performing the play serves as a laboratory for experimenting with sobriety. As each unplanned crisis sent shockwaves through the group, real-time sobriety coaching supported participants in coping with strong emotions and challenging demands. The first question is always, "How do you handle this moment, right now, without turning to substance use?" Answering the question together, in rehearsal, offers rudimentary training in surfacing help from others. A second question, "How is this moment like other moments in your recovery?" helps participants to mentalize the behaviors that will protect healthy sobriety in the future.

Perhaps the strongest message of the play is demonstrated by the action of the story, rather than spoken by a character. The cast insisted on presenting multiple storylines with differing challenges and solutions, varied strategies and philosophies, and a range of resolutions. They wanted a script to show that there is no one answer. Their ability to tolerate the inclusion of ideas in direct conflict with each other, as well as their active participation in realizing those ideas through dramatic presentation, suggests that tolerance and acceptance are two key themes of substance abuse recovery. As the group employed both qualities in the writing of the play, a third element of recovery came clear: hope. The ability to have hope, for oneself and others, is a hallmark of recovery.

Script

PATHS OF THE PRISM

Created by a group in recovery from substance use disorder

2018

CAST OF CHARACTERS

THE GREAT HORN, a God.................................CP2
HERALD, a Healer and Messenger........................Bob
VINCENT, a Visionary and Lover.......................Jeff
MARTHA, a Mother..................................Caitlin
SERIES, her daughter, a lost one...............DT Intern
SAMUEL, her son, lost long ago......................Etan

SETTING: The play takes place between the
                           Heavens and the Earth. The Heavens
                           are home to THE GREAT HORN and all
                           his helpers. Everything there is
                           happy, fun, and blue. Earth is a
                           timeless place where anything can
                           happen. This is a mythical place
                           where people go on epic journeys
                           and face enormous struggles.

Scene 1

(MARTHA is seated working on needlepoint, but
SERIES is in a hurry to start her adventure. She is
storming around the house and packing a bag with
what she needs.)

SERIES

I need the flashlight!

MARTHA

It's in the drawer.

SERIES

Food! I need food!

MARTHA

Peanut butter? In the cabinet.

SERIES

Map! I need a map!

MARTHA

Where are you going?

SERIES

I don't know. I'm lost. I feel like I've always been lost. I've lost my soul. It's been so long, I don't even remember. I have to find my soul, I have to go. I want to show the world the real me, I'm just scared because I feel like people will judge me. Nobody was ever there for me.

MARTHA

I tried my best.

SERIES

But I want to live my life now. I want to change my ways. I'm crying out for help, I have to find my soul.

MARTHA

Please don't go. Can't you just work on yourself here? Stay with me.

SERIES

I can't. I have to go.

MARTHA

I never told you this, but I lost a child before. You had a brother and ... I lost him. He was taken from me. I tried to protect him, I even gave him something magical to protect him ... It doesn't matter, I can't go through it again.

SERIES

Mom, I have to go, I have nothing.

MARTHA

Please stay.

SERIES

I have a map, and I have a pen, I'm gonna mark my way on my journey. I have food, and I have water. I have to go and find what I'm looking for.

MARTHA

Okay, I understand. Here, take this with you. It's a diamond, it will remind you of home.

(SERIES and MARTHA exit in opposite directions.)

Scene 2 : Heaven

(Up in heaven, THE GREAT HORN is holding court. HERALD is hanging on his every word, but VINCENT is standing a little off to the side, unamused. He doesn't buy it.)

HERALD
O Great Horn, what is today's wisdom?

THE GREAT HORN
My children are suffering, it is self-will run riot down there.

HERALD
Yes, I agree, oh great one.

THE GREAT HORN
They are frustrated with what they are trying to accomplish. They have to understand that it's not about them, it's about others.

HERALD
I agree, Great Horn.

THE GREAT HORN
Why are you staring at me?

HERALD
It's the horn. It's just the horn.

THE GREAT HORN
You want to touch it? Touch the horn.

HERALD
Oh! Thank you, Great Horn!

(THE GREAT HORN notices that VINCENT is not participating.)

THE GREAT HORN
Do you want to touch the horn, Vincent? Go ahead, touch the horn.

VINCENT
(heavy sigh)
No. What I want more than anything in the world is for art to be lived, for art to be loved, and consumed with exquisite delight. I look down at them and wish they could consume art and feel the decadence cascading against the soul as if the

warm bosom of passion overflows the brim and spills into the pitcher of ecstasy. As they sip from this pitcher, their desire shall be quenched. If your children are suffering, I'm not sure the great horn is what they need.

                    HERALD
How dare you! Don't be offended, your horniness!

                    THE GREAT HORN
What they need more than anything is for the empty feeling inside to be filled. I know I have seen them conquer lands and kingdoms, and have thousands upon thousands killed and enslaved, all to try to have a purpose. At times, I have regret over the suffering I cause. They have a rage within that feeds off of emptiness, and it just gets deeper and darker. This void can consume them and is the very thing that determines life or death for a large part of the known world.

                    HERALD
Oh yes, I agree Great Horn.

                    VINCENT
I'm not sure I do.

          (A large shofar blows in the distance.)

                    HERALD
The horn, your horniness! Mortal alert!

          (They freeze. SERIES enters below with her bag on
          her back. She is already tired. She's looking for a
          place to sit down. The action in heaven resumes.)

                    THE GREAT HORN
Mortal alert!

                    HERALD
I'll go!

                    VINCENT
No, I'll go.

                    THE GREAT HORN
You both go.

                    HERALD
I won't let you down, oh great one.

VINCENT

I'll show you.

> (They fly down.)

Scene 3

> (We see SERIES. She's covered in dirt and looks
> defeated.)

SERIES

I'm tired ... I'm scared. This is harder than I thought. I'm
like a road runner, I am always running from myself. Let me
just try to sit for a moment.

> (She takes out a notebook and sits on rock to
> write. On the other side of the stage, VINCENT and
> HERALD spot her.)

HERALD

There she is! I got this!

VINCENT

No! If you mess this up, there is no second chance!

HERALD

I'm not going to mess this up! I am the messenger of the Great
Horn; I can't mess this up.

VINCENT

She needs a vision, she needs inspiration.

HERALD

She needs the Great Horn.

> (He turns and appears to her in a blaze of glory.)

HERALD

Behold troubled one! I come from the Great Horn!

> (VINCENT rolls his eyes and walks away.)

SERIES

What the ... ?

HERALD

The answers are within you!

SERIES

You stay right there; don't you take one more step.

> HERALD

No! Listen! I come from the great horniness!

> SERIES

Oh my god, you creep!

> HERALD

No, no! I'm trying to help!

> SERIES

I don't need your help. I'm fine on my own. You stay away!

>> (She scrambles away and leaves her bag. She starts to go around the theater in a loop. VINCENT walks back in.)

> VINCENT

Nice job. Now who's going to tell the Great Horn?

> HERALD

Don't tell the Great Horn! She's just not used to me. I'm here for her, I'll love her through this, and she'll never have to feel like this again. She's worth it, she can do this, she can be happy, she can live again. I'm going after her.

> VINCENT
> (to the audience)

If nothing else, he is determined, and she does deserve the help. I just know there must be some way I can help.

>> (He exits, following them.)

Scene 4

>> (In another part of the Earth, on a city street, the Great Horn enters, but he is in disguise. He has headphones, and a concert t-shirt, and cool kicks. We're not sure if he's THE GREAT HORN, or not. He seems to be someone else. A young man, SAMUEL, enters. He is sad. He's just broken up with another girlfriend. It never seems to work out for him. He thinks he recognizes the Great Horn.)

> SAMUEL

Don't I know you? Dan! Dan Butler, right?

> THE GREAT HORN

Oh, you recognize me?

SAMUEL

Yeah! We worked together at the music studio, Epiphany Records.

THE GREAT HORN

Did we? How are you?

SAMUEL

Well, not great. Another girl just broke up with me. It's like, I'm always looking for someone to complete me, but it never works out.

THE GREAT HORN

That's too bad.

SAMUEL

It's okay. My next plan is to open up a bunch of casinos. I've been dreaming about it since I was 5 when I was on the casino floor, and there were slot machines ringing, coins hitting the metal, and cheers coming from the craps table. I have never set foot in a casino without experiencing that feeling again. It's a vision I've had since I was a kid.

THE GREAT HORN

You were in a casino when you were 5?

SAMUEL

Yeah, I've been on my own for a very long time. What have you been up to? Did you get that job at Epiphany?

THE GREAT HORN

Yeah, I guess you didn't get it.

SAMUEL

No, that's crazy, we were like, at the same level! I guess they just didn't like me.

THE GREAT HORN

Or ... other people just worked harder than you.

SAMUEL

Wow, thanks a lot. Typical.

THE GREAT HORN

Well, good luck man ... you'll need it.

Scene 5

(SERIES is on her journey. HERALD and VINCENT continue to hide but are doing poorly.)

                         SERIES
Quit following me!

                         HERALD
Listen, I know I came on strong, but just hear me out. The
Great Horn is my foundation, and it helps me immensely.

                         SERIES
It's not for me.

                         VINCENT
See? It's not for everyone! Leave that girl alone!

          (HERALD moves to step in front of Series. VINCENT
          pushes him away. This angers HERALD, and he goes in
          for a punch. VINCENT pulls an arrow, strings his
          bow, and as HERALD winds up, the fist and arrow
          collide, shifting the arrow's path into SERIES'S
          ribs.)

                         SERIES
I've been shot!

          (She begins to crawl away. The two gods argue, and
          VINCENT exits. HERALD keeps following SERIES.)

                       Scene 6

          (In another part of the city, on a basketball
          court, THE GREAT HORN enters, but once again, we
          are not exactly sure it's him. This time, he is
          wearing basketball gear, including a headband and
          goggles. He's dribbling and shooting hoops. He's
          great at it. SAMUEL enters even more depressed and
          upset than the last scene. He sees THE GREAT HORN
          playing and remembers that he was great once.)

                         SAMUEL
Aw, hoops!

                     THE GREAT HORN
Wanna take a shot?

                         SAMUEL
Dude, Chris, is that you? We used to play together!

                     THE GREAT HORN
Did we? Take your shot.

>(SAMUEL shoots but misses. THE GREAT HORN snags the rebound.)

SAMUEL

I'm out of practice.

THE GREAT HORN

I'm not. I stick with it, and I work every day.

SAMUEL

Give it here.

>(He shoots again. It's a miss. THE GREAT HORN grabs the rebound.)

THE GREAT HORN

I don't think I remember you.

SAMUEL

Typical. We were the same, but you made the travel team, and then, I don't know . . .

THE GREAT HORN

Take a shot.

>(He throws him the ball. It's the third miss.)

THE GREAT HORN

Man, I ain't got time for this. You got no game, and I'm serious. Go find somewhere else to play.

SAMUEL

No, man! Right now, play me, one on one.

THE GREAT HORN

I don't wanna embarrass you. You already embarrassed yourself.

>(He takes the ball and exits.)

SAMUEL

Give me the ball! Give me the ball! Man, I'm getting so sick and tired of this!

>(He pulls a knife in frustration.)

SAMUEL

This is really pushing me. I feel like I'm on the edge. I give my heart to everything, and nothing works out for me. I could be like anyone else, but I can't make it happen. All these people have done nothing but make something of themselves,

and I know I was better than all of them, and I don't even mean
it like that, but ... why am I here?

> (He looks at the knife.)

Can you help my problems? No, you're just going to make me the
ultimate quitter like they all say I am.

> (He throws the knife toward the park bench. VINCENT
> has been watching the whole game from the bench. He
> knows he can help this guy. He picks up the knife.)

VINCENT

Is this yours?

SAMUEL

Do I know you? You remind me of my art teacher in high school.

VINCENT

You could say I'm an art teacher. You see this beauty out
here? You know, Rome wasn't built in a day.

SAMUEL

I just want it all to happen at once. I just try it and, ugh,
it doesn't work.

VINCENT

You can't have it all now. Oh, be centered young man, before
you lose yourself. Awaken, young man, before you sleep for
eternity. Watch your path so you do not fall upon the jagged
rocks below. Smashed and broken, bloody, bones smeared,
ribs split apart, life leaking out upon the stones. Your
voice, faint as you cry out, but it seems no one can hear you.

SAMUEL

I feel like I'm already there.

VINCENT

Let me give you a gift.

> (He reaches into his coat and takes out a prism.)

This prism is something that I made. It became something
else, something powerful, and I wanted to know what it was
for, and now I know. I'm giving you this power of mine. Find
someone else and give them the gift.

> (SERIES crawls onto the basketball court. HERALD
> is following. He's growing more and more con-
> cerned. Finally, she calls out.)

SERIES

It's too hard. I can't go on. I want to change my ways, I'm crying out for help. Will somebody please help me? Help me!

> (She falls to the ground, as if she's going to die from being shot. Without even thinking about it, SAMUEL stands up, and goes to her. He's able to give his heart to her because now he has the prism.)

SAMUEL

I can help you. Let me help you. Here, take my heart. I'm always giving it away. Maybe it'll do you more good than it's done for me. I have another gift for strength.

> (She takes his heart, and she is restored. She stands up, and she's different.)

SERIES

I feel different. I'm changed. I'm not lost ... I'm found.

HERALD

I did it!!

VINCENT

I did it!!

SERIES

I did it. I asked for help, and I got it, and now that I'm found, I want to go home. I want my mother. I want to go home.

> (She turns to SAMUEL.)

SERIES

Thank you so much. I have nothing to give you. I lost my bag, I lost my way. I have nothing but this diamond. It was supposed to help me get home, but now I think I'll be okay.

SAMUEL

I don't need anything in return. I wish I could go home ... I haven't been home in a long time.

SERIES

Come with me. You look like you could use some help.

HERALD AND VINCENT

We'll help you! We'll protect you! A storm is on the way.

> (THE GREAT HORN creates the sound of thunder from up in heaven. The group comes together under a large protective sheet. The group flocks through

the storm, arriving home. The gods depart, delivering them safely.)

<u>Scene 7</u>

SERIES

Mom? Mom! I'm home!

MARTHA

I'm so happy you're back!

SERIES

Mom, this is my new friend. I almost died, and he gave me his
heart.

SAMUEL

She really did the work, I just came with some guidance.

MARTHA

I knew you would find your way back home. So, did you find what
you were looking for?

SERIES

Yeah, and the diamond you gave me helped to bring us home.

SAMUEL

I don't have anything from my mother, except for this chain.

MARTHA

Let me see that.

SAMUEL

It's missing a piece.

MARTHA

It's missing this.

(She pulls out another diamond.)

MARTHA

This is the stone I should have put on the necklace when I
gave it to my son before I lost him. It fits your chain. I know
you're my son.

SERIES

My brother!

SAMUEL

Mom!

MARTHA

My children! This moment is beyond my wildest dreams. I've always wanted to hold you both, and sing you to sleep.

> (She puts an arm around each one, and sings a lullaby as the gods go back up to the Great Horn.)

Scene 8

HERALD AND VINCENT

We did it!!

THE GREAT HORN

Congratulations.

HERALD

Oh, Great Horn, what is the wisdom of today?

THE GREAT HORN

My plan is that there is no plan. Just come together, and help one another.

HERALD

I agree, Great Horn.
> (He has a tender moment.)

What I've wanted more than anything else in the world is to be just like all the other heavenly helpers. When I went down to Earth, I changed. I didn't always do it perfectly, but I kept going. For me, this was a new way of thinking. A new perspective, and I'm not afraid to show it.

THE GREAT HORN

And you will continue to do my work.

> (He turns to VINCENT)

Will you?

VINCENT

I don't know.

THE GREAT HORN

Don't make this about you!

VINCENT

Haven't I done well?

THE GREAT HORN

It's not about I. It's about everybody. Follow the flow, don't make it about you. Find a path, and follow it.

VINCENT

What is my path? I've been told to follow my heart, but if I do it myself, I don't know how it will turn out.

THE GREAT HORN

You are a visionary, Vincent. Look up. Look forward. What do you see?

VINCENT

It's the path. I see the path.

THE GREAT HORN

Don't just talk about miracles, show me one.

(VINCENT begins to walk down the path.)

(END OF PLAY)

Discussion Questions

1 CoATT participants must identify themselves as "in active recovery." What evidence of active recovery is found in the script? Are there instructions for living that support an active recovery?
2 This group chose a title that suggests multiple paths in recovery. Each individual in the group was intent on telling their own story of recovery, in addition to answering the CoATT Question as a group. Track the dramatic arc of each character as a single dramatic line, then draw parallels to recovery between each.
3 Do you think that all the characters end in a state that parallels "active recovery"? In what ways? How does each journey show the need to find recovery? Why might one group be committed to showing moments of struggle and challenge when another group might choose to focus on lessons from inside active recovery?
4 Many phrases in this play are taken directly from 12-step recovery literature or are commonly heard slogans from 12-step meetings, yet no overt reference is made to 12-step recovery. Instead, the Great Horn and Herald are presented as orthodox or canonized wisdom. Describe the dramatic tension between orthodox thinking and artistic exploration that exists in the play.
5 The Great Horn appears to Samuel in three different personas. What is the significance of Samuel interacting with the Great Horn but continuing on his journey toward suicidality?
6 Describe the relationship between Vincent, Herald, and the Great Horn. How does this relationship depict relationships between individuals who are all living in active recovery?

Reference List

Alcoholics Anonymous. (2002). *The big book* (4th ed.). Alcoholics Anonymous World Services. https://www.aa.org/the-big-book

Alcoholics Anonymous. (2021, June 23). *A.A. Preamble*. Alcoholics Anonymous World Services. https://www.aa.org/sites/default/files/literature/smf-92_en.pdf

Capra, F. (1946). *It's a wonderful life* [Film]. Liberty Films.

Kopelovich, S. L., & Turkington, D. (2021). Remote CBT for psychosis during the COVID-19 pandemic: challenges and opportunities. *Community Mental Health Journal, 57*: 30–34. 10.1007/s10597-020-00718-0

Landy, R. J. (1994). *Drama therapy: Concepts, theories and practices* (2nd ed.). Charles C. Thomas. https://psycnet.apa.org/record/1994-98841-000

Pendzik, S. (2016). The dramaturgy of autobiographical therapeutic performance. In S. Pendzik, R. Emunah, & D. R. Johnson (Eds.), *The self in performance: autobiographical, self-revelatory, and autoethnographic forms of therapeutic theatre* (pp. 55–69). Palgrave Macmillan. 10.1057/978-1-137-53593-1

Chapter 8

Future Directions

As we approach the conclusion of this book, we continue to learn through and about the model we have created. We ask: What is the mechanism of transformation at work in the CoATT model? How does this process operate across such disparate groups? Where does change happen within the seven movements of a CoATT production? How do each of the operating principles drive recovery?

CoATT is built around the question: What is a theme of recovery you want to create a play about to strengthen your recovery and share with an audience? This grounding opens the door to as many future directions as there are groups in recovery. The participants in treatment for aphasia presented a wide range of answers to this prompt. Initially, the group wished to demystify the condition with messages as simple as, "We are the same people we were before the trauma," or, "We are not stupid, we have aphasia." Later they began to delve into concepts that reflect the challenges of living in recovery, such as "parenting a teenager in recovery requires an extra layer of firmness and patience." Can CoATT plays take on a teaching or skill-training message that empowers members of a specific recovery community to help newer members connect to that community?

People living with chronic mental illnesses like schizophrenia may use a wellness recovery model that acknowledges the presence of a disease and stresses the maintenance of a standard of care. These groups offer the opportunity to explore recovery that is separated from the concept of improvement or self-help. They may be uniquely poised to explore a recovery based on self-acceptance and de-stigmatization. Some approaches to wellness for chronic mental illness insist on radical acceptance of a wider range of sensory input than is typically experienced. Can CoATT plays created by groups with this definition of recovery offer insight into the benefits of living with schizophrenia, for example? The power to shift perspective, in aphasia treatment and beyond, could have a great impact on the medical model of treatment.

Two of the operating principles that drive CoATT open the door to future directions. The first focuses the work on the CoATT question and

DOI: 10.4324/9781003161608-9

exploration, and the second locates CoATT at a specific time in treatment. Thus far, CoATT has been used with cohorts that are poised to step down from more intensive treatment settings and live in active recovery. Group members must be able to articulate a definition of recovery and find enough common ground with fellows to support the work of playmaking. That kind of abstract thinking and flexibility may need some scaffolding, and the work of the Rehearsal phase serves as a laboratory for experimentation. Participants learn to share their worldview, to express and activate their feelings about diagnosis and recovery in a group setting where the impact of their actions adds meaning and value to the play without suffering real-world consequences for their risk-taking. Rehearsal is a safe enough space to explore, where there is room to rewrite, reconfigure, and try it all again.

This is shown to be of enormous value in conceptions of recovery that are grounded in "then/now" thinking. One commonality between eating disorder recovery groups and substance use disorder groups was the perception that stopping a behavior (binge/restrict cycling, or use of a substance) creates a new reality for the individual in recovery. For both groups, control was an essential feature in the suffering before recovery. For both groups, the loss of that control made it difficult to move beyond concrete reality-based statements. Negotiating play, creative expression, and imaginary reality as means for creating connection can be challenging; yet isolation has been shown to be (literally) deadly in recovery. Playmaking in a group process may delay the isolation but is also shown to foster the skill of making connections with others. One limitation of the CoATT model is that it may simply extend treatment time before the inevitable return to "the regular world."

Our contention is that a CoATT production supports a Launch into "the regular world," providing key preparation to thrive in recovery. Each of the plays presented here, and the group processes that led to them, have commonalities and differences in content, style, and even (perhaps) quality. To understand the mechanisms of change at work in CoATT, it's important to focus on the common features that are reinforced through the core principles (Figure 8.1).

The model above shows Growth in Recovery plotted against the movements of the CoATT model. During Recruitment and Discovery, the group is working toward safety and containment. We acknowledge a step-down from treatment that often precedes CoATT recruitment as a stepping *into* new relationships and a new level of recovery. These meetings buffer the adjustment by creating a healthy group to support individual recovery.

Generation, Intensive, and Rehearsal sessions then allow participants to explore new roles in a recovery setting, while practicing the new skills needed to build connection. In these meetings, they practice working together, problem-solving, challenging each other, frustration tolerance, and mentalizing a different future or outcome. They may play through mistakes or poor choices without suffering real-world consequences. Working in metaphor

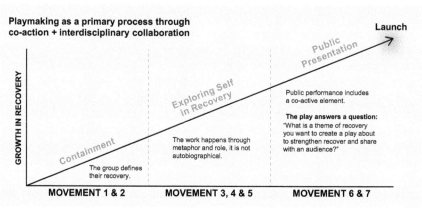

Figure 8.1 The CoATT Model Mechanisms of Transformation.

moves them away from concrete, autobiographical, rigid thinking and conditions. They play at recovery and play at connection with others.

During Performance and Launch, the CoATT model stresses recovery behaviors and healthy connections with the community at large. Co-action in the creative space of playmaking blurs into the co-creation of a new reality in recovery.

This chart outlines the progress of the CoATT model, identifying the order of operations for making a play and theorizing a connection between playmaking and recovery. The manualized order allows for replicability that will in turn allow for a study of the effectiveness of CoATT as an intervention in recovery. Such studies will add to the evidence base on the impact CoATT productions have on the psychological functioning and well-being of participants (i.e., outcome research).

However, recent research in creative arts therapies (CAT) has focused more specifically on studies of the *mechanisms of change* that underpin a CAT intervention (de Witte et al., 2021). A recent scoping review considered 67 studies to pinpoint therapeutic factors at work in CATs, joint factors across the disciplines, and common factors shared with most other psychotherapy approaches (DeWitt et al., 2021). In addition to the useful categorization of therapeutic factors, terminology used in change process research has been clarified through this work.

As a foundational component of this effort, the North American Drama Therapy Association (NADTA) research committee opened an important discussion exploring "the specific and key elements that contribute to the practice of drama therapy; the observable building blocks thought to create dynamic conditions for change" (Frydman et al., 2022 p.4). Building on Jones

(2016) the research team implemented a Delphi study to identify a revised set of seven core processes in drama therapy, including dramatic projection, dramatic play, dramatic embodiment, multi-dimensional relationship, active witnessing, embodiment, and distancing.

With these operationalized terms the field is set to track a sequence of the presence of core processes, leading to technicisms of change, which facilitate desired outcomes. As relevant to CoATT, future studies could examine which core processes create the conditions for mechanisms of change to arise and facilitate desirable outcomes.

The chart below borrows from both studies to theoretically describe the mechanism of change most specific to CoATT. We believe that the CoATT Movements outline a sequence of events and processes that explain how participants change. Against the line of CoATT production, we have charted the common factors of psychotherapy at work using language from de Witte et al. (2021) and shown the core processes of drama therapy manualized into the model using the language from Frydman et al. (2022) and Jones (2016). The chart calls special attention to Yalom and Leszcz (2020) 11 common factors for therapeutic change in group psychotherapy.

We think the most unique element of CoATT is the use of the life-drama connection, particularly in the group and public settings of rehearsal and performance. One promising line of drama therapy research might be the study of how the core processes of drama therapy in CoATT facilitate the change delivered by life-drama connection. Other researchers may choose to focus on one Movement or exercise in CoATT and research how mediating variables such as playmaking impact common factors of psychotherapy. We hope our manualized model affords clear locations for many CAT studies.

CoATT's unique benefits could be valuable in a variety of therapeutic settings. But adapting it for them, while maintaining fidelity to the model we have laid out in this book, may present some challenges. A few examples below illustrate opportunities for growth, alongside questions that future researchers would have to answer when deploying CoATT in a new field.

For example, could CoATT be applied to a group or setting that centers treatment, rather than recovery – that is, where there is no internal, harmful behavior to overcome? Perhaps. Imagine a CoATT process for adult survivors of childhood sexual abuse who are well along in their individual recovery journeys. The nature of the wounds being carried from abuse and trauma can be such that therapeutic work may, at best, be able to support living better with the knowledge of what has happened. This is different from a changed behavior of moving away from substance use or an eating disorder. Would CoATT, in this context, be offered by a therapist with a specialized practice? Could it substitute as a phase of group therapy for groups focused on a particular type of traumatic experience?

Can this model be placed at a different point in the recovery journey? Again, perhaps. Imagine CoATT becoming a featured model within a residential treatment protocol, supporting early work toward recovery. One challenge might be determining how an inpatient program can welcome a public audience, as CoATT requires, in service of reconnection.

Can CoATT be used to directly address recovery from issues of oppression? Maybe. Consider a group of individuals who are seeking recovery from harmful internalized messages of fat-phobia. CoATT may be valuable here – if the participants could find a common theme around which to answer the CoATT Question.

Although we don't know the answers to these questions, we would support thoughtful exploration of new directions if the six principles of the model guide the effort. As the hypotheticals above illustrate, that is easier said than done. But the challenges are likely not insurmountable.

Online CoATT performances taught us that the theatre itself is always adapting to circumstances. While the Covid-19 pandemic morphs into the next phases it will leave some permanent changes to many aspects of our lives. Telemedicine and teletherapy have become normalized, and for some models, expanded treatment delivery. CoATT explored presenting plays online and found that some adaptations were truly beneficial to the participants. Removing the need to commute for rehearsals or memorize lines opens participation to many people with chronic conditions. Results of those studies show that making connections with others remained a positive outcome of the protocol. What other adapted forms of playmaking might adopt a CoATT approach? In any setting where isolation is a threat to recovery, the model might be adapted to fit the needs of the group.

CoATT must, therefore, remain interdisciplinary. A clear understanding of presenting issues is critical to imagining recovery in a meaningful way. Drama therapists may lead the way in playmaking as a primary process, and participants may lead the way toward definitions of recovery, but clinical expertise on medical, psychological, and interpersonal traumas will always benefit CoATT productions. Building these interdisciplinary relationships begins by ensuring people with different expertise understand the options for, and benefits of, collaborating on a CoATT production. This book, and manualized form, aims to advance that goal – by mitigating the skepticism, or unfamiliarity, that might intimidate colleagues from other disciplines.

The CoATT Model began as a simple project, like many plays, with two clinicians saying to each other, "Let's put on a show." We were surrounded by riches in resources, most particularly with the group of participants assembled. This group had all completed treatment at a nationally recognized eating disorder center. All of them were healthy, thanks in large part to the conception of recovery they worked to discover in treatment. All of them had more than a year of practice in drama therapy, and all under the direction of Laura. The entire group was poised on the brink of re-entry into the community and deeply committed to their own recovery. Each had an individual sense that helping support others would be implicit in their own successful launch. There was considerable enthusiasm to match the considerable talent. Everyone agreed that they were ready for a step beyond the drama therapy group: they wanted to do a scripted play.

Laura had developed internationally recognized expertise in the treatment of eating disorders. She had the support of the institution and not just goodwill. The facility provided after-hours access to rehearsal space, as well as financial support for the public presentation. Everyone involved in that initial production, *I Remember Justine*, shared the highest standards for both treatment and production.

The success of the initial play seemed like the "magic of the theater" and the "beauty of drama therapy." It also suggested that the process could and should be repeated. That group did so, including many new members in a new cast and new production. This afforded us the chance to begin replicating the approach in a manualized fashion. News of our success traveled, and with no effort on our part, other clinicians with expertise in different populations asked to participate in productions using "the model." It was the dedication of a speech pathology department that offered us an incredibly strong group of participants to explore recovery from medical trauma. It was a colleague in social work who offered access to an outpatient treatment facility and an associated halfway house that were looking to energize recovery from substance use disorder.

With each group, we expanded and refined the key concepts of the model, particularly the focus on active recovery and the timing of the intervention. The process and progress of playmaking became more explicit, leading to an easy step-by-step series of meetings and rehearsals. Ultimately, this process led to the manual contained in this book. This enormous amount of work all took place on a volunteer basis, supported by generous donations and optimistic underwriting.

Working after hours and during everyone's spare time, however, puts limits on what work can be offered and how much access we can provide for participants. It limits where the work can go, and how we can train people to do the work while emulating the highest standard. Educational institutions can give some focus to the work, but always at the expense of another model, program, or approach. Treatment centers are built on profit-making models and have limits on development funding. Participants confront the real-world demands on their time and their money, which may prevent them from paying to produce the work.

The need to associate this work with treatment centers, and to formalize the relationship between payers in the health care system and practitioners of the model, has become acute. The future of the work depends on funding. So, we look to other successful models that are supported in the health care ecosystem. These models, like cognitive behavioral therapy, are certified as evidence-based treatments.

Evidence-based treatments (EBTs) are still a relatively new concept in the overarching history of mental health, with an explosion of interest beginning in the 1990s. The practice of EBTs took root in the medical professions and began to inform and influence other professions, including the field of psychotherapy (Cook et al., 2017).

As Landy made clear, though, psychoanalysis and psychotherapy have been informed by the sensibility of the artist and were further defined through the lens of relational approaches (1996). As a result, for drama therapists and creative arts therapist, EBT may not sit as comfortably in our conception of the work. For some, words associated with EBT, like "manualization," have a bad reputation in the world of psychotherapy and the arts and may even engender misconceptions. Treatment providers may be frustrated when they believe that their work is devalued without an evidence-based certification. Self-expression may resist the limitations that come with all forms of research. The fear that manualization equates to rigidity threatens the use of interpretation and artistic expertise. Manuals for treatment may seem to be merely cookbooks that replace clinical experience and judgment with measurements and process steps. Some even believe that the focus on standardized outcomes in EBT practice means discarding the client's needs.

Another objection may relate to the ever-changing nature of CoATT productions and treatment. Therapeutic theatre is a powerful modality, and performance is transformative. The CoATT model gets refined and enhanced in production, as well as after production. So, why bother to create a manual and seek the designation of being an EBT?

The simple answer is that adopting EBT practices may expand the availability of CoATT, given the financial realities of clinical practice. If a treatment isn't considered evidence-based, then managed health care in the United States withholds reimbursement. Indeed, Laura has seen clients denied access to the forms of therapy that she heard helped them on similar grounds. Our colleagues working in both substance-use counseling and community health care have all faced similar denials. For those patients in the early stages of active recovery, these are the moments where relapse is most likely to strike and is arguably the most destructive, and the missed opportunity can be devastating. For the clinicians who treat them, the dynamic is deflating. Evidence-based therapy recognition for CAT models like CoATT may make a significant difference in positive outcomes.

We find that revisiting the definition of EBT can be helpful in reminding us that the goal of an EBT is rooted in the desire to best serve individuals by creating just such outcomes. The term "evidence-based" was first formally defined by Sackett et al. (1996) as the "conscientious, explicit, and judicious use of current best evidence in making decisions about the care of individual patients." At the heart, the goal is to support practitioners in choosing treatments that are shown to support their client's care, offering ethical and thoughtful practice. Over time, EBT has expanded to also include "consideration of patients preferences, actions, clinical state, and circumstances" (Cook et al., 2017, p. 537). So, despite the negative reputation EBTs have among creative arts therapists who view them as overly outcome-driven, EBTs, at their core, are built on honoring a collaborative experience between practitioner and client, as well as on choosing treatments that have a strong evidence base to support that choice.

What dictates a strong evidence base? Critically, EBT practice looks to a wide variety of evidence and does not limit itself to purely quantitative work. Instead, most individuals are surprised to learn that evidence in EBT practice can entail a wide variety of research, from meta-analyses, randomized controlled trials (RCTs), effectiveness studies, and process studies, to high-level forms of qualitative research that include single-case reports, systematic case studies and clinical observation (Cook et al., 2017).

The field of drama therapy is certainly not short of case studies and meaningful clinical observations. But other forms of quantitative research (RCTs and effectiveness studies) are lacking in our field (Armstrong et al., 2019). Therapeutic theatre needs a manual that supports such standardization, one that has strong fidelity measures to accompany it.

We are currently making our way through the RCT quagmire and have seen firsthand how valuable manualization can be. Due to the pandemic, our first RCT converted to a multi-play trial under the direction of Dr. Xiaduo Fan. Dr. Fan, a psychiatrist at UMass Mind, is passionate about using the arts to help individuals with serious mental illnesses. He knows that alternative forms of treatment are needed to support recovery, and initially reached out with the hope of building a manual. When he found out one already existed, it expedited our collaboration. With this support, we applied and were awarded a National Endowment for the Arts Grant to produce five plays over 30 months with individuals diagnosed with schizophrenia. A large National Institute for Health grant application was submitted in the winter of 2023, in hopes of pursuing a multi-city RCT with the model and individuals with serious and persistent mental illnesses (SPMI). A grant of this level was, in part, made possible due to having a manual. We can offer granting agencies an assurance of fidelity while supporting participants in the trials with the flexibility that yields meaningful progress.

We envision a change. We are optimistic that the model gives a way for formal treatment centers to build relationships with their identified community and clients through using the CoATT model. We imagine a world in which CoATT is standard care and is accessible to anyone who identifies as being in active recovery. We dare to see the model as a tool, covered by insurance, so that professionals, institutions, and participants can all benefit. We imagine communities loving local theatre with participants in productions, plays that are opening conversations, and centers of activity that can provide resources and that can destigmatize mental health treatment. We see a lot of strong recovery.

In order to do this, numerous practitioners must join us in building an evidence base for the model. We must find clinicians with expertise in recovery populations who view themselves as being in "active recovery." Using the manual, and training in the model from both roles that facilitate the work, can create even more opportunities for clinical trials. Perhaps funding can be found to conduct any of the types of research listed above that build on a claim to EBT. Studies in eating disorder treatment, substance use disorders, aphasia, or schizophrenia will build on the evidence base that exists. Once we have enough studies, we hope to apply for EBT approval in the next five to seven years.

Most important is that we continue to forge ahead in creating multiple ways to support individuals in recovery through sustainable and accessible means. Recovery doesn't happen in treatment centers; it happens in people's lives, relationships, communities, and connections.

Reference List

Armstrong, C. R., Frydman, J. S., & Rowe, C. (2019). A snapshot of empirical drama therapy research: Conducting a general review of the literature. *GMS Journal of Arts Therapies*, *1*(2). 10.3205/jat000002

Cook, S. C., Schwartz, A. C., & Kaslow, N. J. (2017). Evidence-based psychotherapy: Advantages and challenges. *Neurotherapeutics*, *14*(3): 537–545. 10.1007/s13311-017-0549-4

De Witte, M., Orkibi, H., Zarate, R., Karkou, V., Sajnani, N., Malhotra, B., ... & Koch, S. C. (2021). From therapeutic factors to mechanisms of change in the creative arts therapies: A scoping review. *Frontiers in Psychology*, 2525.

Frydman, J. S., Cook, A., Armstrong, C. R., Rowe, C., & Kern, C. (2022). The drama therapy core processes: A Delphi study establishing a North American perspective. *The Arts in Psychotherapy*, *80*: 101939.

Jones, P. (2016). How do dramatherapists understand client change?: A review of the 'core processes' at work. *Routledge international handbook of dramatherapy*, 77–91.

Landy, R. J. (1996). *Persona and performance: The meaning of role in drama, therapy, and everyday life*. Guilford. https://psycnet.apa.org/record/1994-97043-000

Sackett, D. L., Rosenberg, W. M. C., Gray, J. A. M., Haynes, R. B., & Richardson, W. S. (1996). Evidence based medicine: What it is and what it isn't. *BMJ*, *312*: 71–72. 10.1136/bmj.312.7023.71

Yalom, I. D., & Leszcz, M. (2020). *The theory and practice of group psychotherapy*. Basic books.

Appendices

Appendix A: Partnership Checklist

The pre-process checklist is a tool that can be used when a team of CoATT practitioners is collaborating with a new organization or intuitional partnership. The checklist is not exhaustive, and all elements may also not be applicable. It is a way to start a dialogue about some of the unique aspects that can arise when a group of an organization is taking on this work for the first time.

1 Is there an official definition of recovery that your institution enforces?
2 What is your code of behavior for patients, clients, or participants? Do they have a treatment agreement?
3 What is your code of conduct for staff members, including licensed personnel, unlicensed support staff, and facility workers?
4 Do you have rules regarding vendor relationships?
5 Are there guidelines or restrictions on materials the group can use?
6 For staff members (including licensed personnel, unlicensed support staff, and facility workers) who are involved in the CoATT process, how will supervision be handled?
7 How will communication between CoATT practitioners and institutional staff happen and what material do you expect to share?
8 What are the rules around communicating with the participants, including phone, social media, and personal contact? What about after-hours contact? How are patient/staff boundaries delineated?
9 What is the expected plan for documentation?
10 Do both parties have clearly articulated expectations for workload, compensation, expenses, and reimbursement?
11 How are liability issues handled?
12 What is the escalation policy?

Appendix B: Production Checklist

Production Check-List

These tasks are completed during the Rehearsal movement during the appropriate weeks depending on production pacing. Some productions may be fortunate enough to have a therapeutic stage manager who may work with participants to facilitate these steps in a therapeutic manner. Additionally, some roles may be filled by previous participants.

Task	Who will complete	Date completed
Finding people participants trust to run lines with outside of rehearsal		
Memorizing lines		
Listing out who to invite to the play		
Supporting cast in inviting people to the play		
Deciding on costumes		
Buying or constructing costumes		
Deciding on props		
Buying or constructing props		
Set design		
Set construction		
Creation of a poster for production		
Creation of a playbill for production		
Publicizing the public performance		
Lighting for stage		
Sound for Stage		
Greeting for production		
Pre-show event (tables, raffles, psychoeducation, etc)		
After show refreshments		

Notes

Figure 9.1 Production Checklist.

Appendix C: Rehearsal Report

Rehearsal Report

Show:

Location _____

Day/Time _____ Date _____

Completed by _____

Rehearsal Start	
Rehearsal End	
Next Rehearsal	
Rehearsal Schedule	

Attendance _____ Late _____ Absent _____

Scenery:	**Sound:**

Lighting:	**Costumes:**

Properties:	**Stage Management:**

Script Changes:

Figure 9.2 Rehearsal Report.

Appendix D: Worksheets for Practitioners

```
┌─────────────────────────────────────────────────────────────┐
│ Content Notes:                                              │
│                                                             │
│                                                             │
│                                                             │
│                                                             │
│                                                             │
└─────────────────────────────────────────────────────────────┘

┌─────────────────────────────────────────────────────────────┐
│ Recovery Notes:                                            │
│                                                             │
│                                                             │
│                                                             │
│                                                             │
│                                                             │
└─────────────────────────────────────────────────────────────┘

┌─────────────────────────────────────────────────────────────┐
│ Rehearsal Notes:                                           │
│                                                             │
│                                                             │
│                                                             │
│                                                             │
│                                                             │
└─────────────────────────────────────────────────────────────┘

┌─────────────────────────────────────────────────────────────┐
│ Field Notes:        □ Descriptive  □ Interpretative  □ Reflexive │
│                                                             │
│                                                             │
│                                                             │
│                                                             │
└─────────────────────────────────────────────────────────────┘
```

Figure 9.3 Practitioner Note Page.

Miscellaneous/Additional Notes:

Figure 9.4 Miscellaneous/Additional Notes Page.

Appendix E: Sample CoATT Semi-Structured Individual Interview

Co-Active Therapeutic Theatre

Semi-Structured Interview Protocol for individual interviews or focus groups.

1   Tell me about your experience of being a part of the CoActive Therapeutic Theatre group.
2   In what ways, if any, do you believe this project supported your active recovery?
3   What benefits, if any, did you take away from the process?
4   This process is called "co-active" because participants are "co-actively" partnering with the facilitators, each other, and the audience. Was this your experience, and if so, did this affect your experience of the process?
5   Your group answered the question "What is a theme of recovery you want to work on in service of your recovery?" Your group selected the theme _____. Tell me more about what it meant for you to work on this theme.
6   What was it like for your words to be included in the script of the play?
7   You performed for a public audience; what did it mean for you to perform for this group?
8   What was most challenging for you in this process?
9   What was most joyful for you in this process?
10 How is working on a CoATT production different from just group talk therapy, if at all?
11 Anything else you would like to speak to regarding the Co-Active Therapeutic Theatre model?

Note: In groups that we have ongoing grounded theory data on, we incorporate those findings into a focus group. For example, one finding for clients with eating disorders is that the process helps build community, so the question asked is:

• "In what ways, if any, did this process help you build community?"
• Probe: If yes, how does building community support your recovery?

Appendix F: Sample Strengths and Resources Worksheet

Strengths that I currently have	Strengths that I am working on developing, and how I am actively working on it	A strength I hope to have at the end of this production and how I might use the theater process to help

Reasons why I am recovering	People I know I can count on as a resource	Someone new in this production I want to get to know (add their phone number below)

Figure 9.5 Sample Strengths and Resources Worksheet.

Index